Make Your Way to Being an Herbalist

Written By Kathy Eich

The Pocket Herbalist Series, Book I

Acknowledgements

I would like to thank my editor, Talitha Cushman. Her sharp eye, keen intellect, hard work, and diligence helped me draw to a close a project that has taken years.

Thanks, also, to my sister, Victoria Gritton, for putting together a book cover that is modern and unique, and to photographer Jeff Weyer for the Saturday afternoon photo shoot. Jeff took the author photo for the printed edition.

Thank you to my husband, John Eich, for his unwavering support and encouragement, and for his willingness to master the art of formatting a Word-to-Kindle doc despite tediousness.

Last but not least, thank you to my kids, students and clients who, over the course of the last 18 + years, have helped to shape my personal voice and philosophy around the practice and study of herbal medicine. One can learn about herbs in books and in the wild, but it takes a community to train an herbalist.

Table of Contents

horseradish, licorice, linden, lobelia, marshmallow root, milky oat seed, motherwort, osha, passionflower, peppermint, plantain leaf, sage, skullcap, thyme, usnea, yarrow

Chapter 12 - Infused Oil *Materia medica*

Plants Covered: arnica, calendula, chaparral, comfrey root or leaf, mullein flower, plantain, sage, St. John's wort

Chapter 13 - Essential Oil *Materia medica*

Essential Oils Covered: cinnamon, clary sage, *Eucalyptus globulus*, frankincense, geranium, lavender, lemongrass, mandarin, vetiver, ylang ylang

Bibliography

Introduction

"We have only to use our intelligence to realize that we...have a constantly replenishing supply of lifesaving remedies all around us. Using leaves, barks, flowers, and berries, using earth, fire and water, people accumulated over the centuries a great body of natural healing lore...being remembered again."

Nature's Children, by Juliette de Bairacli Levy

A little over one hundred years ago, here in North America, the use of plant medicines was commonplace. There was a certain philosophy and preparedness around healing, using plants as the vehicle to cure. And if you didn't know which one to reach for, your friend, neighbor, or the town herbalist did.

With an idea and plant material in hand, a trip to the kitchen would yield a concoction to sooth the day's woe, be it headache, heartache, or belly ache. Alive were the medicines, and active was the community that supported each other in healing.

Back then, the local herbalist was a constant in communities. Their role was vital, as they carried the traditions handed to them by their ancestors to provide the same support, education, and medicines to their towns.

By the early 20th century, the seeds of modern ideas, well propagated, led to the decline of herbal medicine. Contributing factors were the invention of penicillin and the popularity of processed foods. Despite the fact that fewer people were using plants as medicines, some traditionalists respectfully tended the old ways. Native Americans, Appalachian healers, the Curanderos from Mexico, and Chinese immigrates were a few of the small and quietly practicing bands of people. They were typically isolated or separate from the inner circle of society, segregated by cultural differences to maintain a support system of like-mindedness.

But these good keepers of old ways were not alone. They were joined by others in America, whose strong and notable voices kept the torch of plant medicine burning in the mainstream, like the Eclectic Doctors of the 19th and early 20th century. These good doctors considered herbalism to be the heart of medicine and believed that a body's vital force needed live medicines. Their documentation and literature has endured and is the backbone of Western herbalism today.

As time passed, herbalism withstood some dark decades. But still, enough people were moved to remember and keep the practice alive. Their revivals were intended to balance current social trends and empower people. Many of those from the 60's and 70's still practice today to improve and make more credible the practice of herbalism. They are familiar names: Matt Wood, David Winston, Amanda McQuade Crawford, Aviva Romm, David Hoffman, Rosemary Galdstar, Jeanne Rose, Susan Weed, and the late Michael Moore.

While their ideas are not understood by all, each of these individuals has a mission. Their collective beliefs, bold spirits, and care for humanity fortifies a movement that they view as a healing right. A movement that, despite bad press or the inability of studies to scientifically prove why plants work, has kept people's curiosity piqued.

And now, nearly 100 years since its decline, herbalism is strong. The revitalization of plants as medicines boasts a community of herbalists, allopathic physicians, traditional advocates, and folk healers that has grown to amass itself in the hundreds of thousands globally. You see plant people almost everywhere. And they are showing the world the many ways that grassroots herbalism grows by actively leading their communities through teaching, writing, starting businesses, practicing, and handing old wisdoms to their children and grandchildren. They are spreading this infectious art, because once a plant heals for you, you pass the word. Herbs do work!

Through my work in writing, teaching, seeing clients, and owning an herb store, I have learned and observed many things. One of the most important things I have learned is a catalyst for this book. It is that herbalism is not just about the plants. People play an equally important role. Plants work best when individuals are empowered to use them properly and when there is a strong community to share and support the use of herbs. It is our responsibility as educators to teach the foundations of use that forge the plant-to-person-to-community relationship.

Make Your Way to Being an Herbalist is my contribution to this growing field. As a book and resource, it is a companion to the beginning herbal enthusiast. It covers the basic philosophy needed to learn herbalism and aromatherapy, as well as clear instructions for safely and effectively making and using herb and aromatherapy products for acute conditions. For practical use and example, there are also sample plant formulas for the conditions listed, and a *Materia medica* covering essential oils, plants for internal use, and plants for infused oils.

The practice of herbalism is an art. Color, variation, tempo, and timbre are different for every user and practitioner of plant medicine. My intention is that this book helps you carve your own path and find your own voice in this ever-growing field. May the plants be with you on your path.

Section 1

Philosophy and Making: Chapters 1-7

Chapter 1

Herbalism

Getting Started

Being an herbalist means being ambidextrous. In one week, you may find yourself treating bee stings, formulating for bronchitis, or mixing up a remedy for insomnia. To support this flexibility, it's important to cultivate an understanding of how plants interface with people and the maladies that affect them. That takes time, study, thought, work experience, and observation.

At times, the amount of information we feel we need to know can be overwhelming, and advanced and beginning students alike will ask, "Will I ever feel like I know enough?" My reply is, "Of course you will. You probably already do." And then I tell them this: "Matt Wood, one of the leading herbalists of our time, tells his students, 'If you know how to use one plant, and use it effectively and well, then you are a Master Herbalist.'"

In its simplicity, this essential piece of advice reminds us that everyone began somewhere. And that looking on the bright side of what you know feeds your sense of accomplishment, thereby inspiring you forward. It also denotes, with grace, that you don't need to know everything to be an accomplished herbalist, and that it is important to remember your limits.

Speaking of limits, we all have them. In this day and age, herbalism is complicated by many things – chronic disease, modern diet, lifestyle choices, and prescription drugs with their interactions. These can make recommending and using plants internally very difficult.

What's my advice for dealing with these issues when you are a beginner? Focus on the following things in your quest for knowledge and experience:

> ➢ Learn how to use a few plants instead of 20 or 100.
> ➢ Find plants that are already growing in nature around you, and/or grow them.

- Learn how to make the medicines, and learn well. You will receive instructions for this in the chapters to come.
- Use the few things you're working with on yourself and your family to gain experience.
- Observe and take note of when you use a plant and whether it does or doesn't work. Take note of who used it, what the reaction was, and meditate on possible reasons for the outcome.
- Study and work to understand and remember energetic terms (words that outline how herbs work). You will be able to read and understand high quality herbal literature and teachers if you do so.
- Begin to learn plant-to-person interface with tonic plants by recommending remedies for first aid and acute illness.
- Know your limits and who to go to when you're in over your head. Saying, "I don't know," is a great answer. It doesn't mean that you've failed.

Ways to Use Plants Medicinally

If you've read this far or were drawn to this book at all, you know that herbalism is the practice of using plants as medicines. But what you may not know is the many ways we use them. When most people think of herbs as medicines, they imagine ingesting capsules and drinking teas, some knowing what a tincture is.

But therapeutic plant use is even more comprehensive than ingestion. Because when we use a plant, we're not simply fixing a problem. We're affecting mucous, blood, bile, water, eliminatory organs, nervous system, hormonal firings, and our emotional and spiritual bodies, just to name a few.

Eliciting a reaction can be as simple as drinking a cup of tea, but it is also bigger. It is intention and faith that something will move. It is leaving our expectations behind and putting hope in its place. And it involves many ways to use plants, both externally and internally. Here is a fairly comprehensive list of applications.

- Burning herbs
- Full body, hand, or foot tea baths
- Tea infusions of aromatic plants poured over hot rocks in sweat lodges
- Essential oil inhalation or room diffusion (aromatherapy)

- Topical application of essential oil products, including massage, bath, hand and foot rubs
- Using infused oils in salves for topical healing
- Internal consumption of plant infusions in water as tea, alcohol or glycerin as tinctures, cooking, honey or vinegar, and ground to be put into capsules
- Sleeping with essential oils or plant pillows for insomnia or dream work
- Carrying plants as a talisman for power and protection
- Observing and drawing plants
- Gardening and growing plants
- The act of making medicine
- Crafting with plants
- Reading and writing about plants

Most people don't realize that noticing a plant, reading about it, or drawing it can elicit a healthy change, but it can. I've seen it happen. If you were to begin drawing or reading about a plant, which one would it be?

How Do We Decide What Plants to Use?

Beginning Concepts for Acute Illness Formulation:

There are many things an herbalist will consider when choosing the right plant or group of plants (formula) for a person. Some of them are quite complicated. In the beginning, there are a few basic principles that one can focus on as they practice. As you grow your understanding and application of them, you can delve into concepts that are more advanced. The details of application will be further explained and explored in Section 2 of this book.

- Know your symptoms and the energetics (plant actions) needed to deal with them. Whether you have a spastic cough or nasal congestion, there is a plant for it.
- Pick your plant based on the affinity of the herb to the illness and system of the body affected. Do you have a virus that affects the lungs? Pick a plant that has an affinity or effect on the lungs.
- Is your cough wet or dry, and are your lungs feeling hot or cold? Chose plants that have the proper quality (warming, cooling, moistening, or drying). Do you have an acute respiratory illness? That's generally a sign that your immune

system needs warming. So pick an herb with warming qualities.

Examples of Intermediate to Advanced Concepts:

I'm briefly mentioning these ideas, but don't worry too much about them now. They will be further explained in more advanced texts.

> - Affinity of herb-to-organ system through energetics – the four qualities and their degrees of hot, cold, dry, wet, and the two tensions, stimulation and relaxation
> - Affinity of herb-to-disease or symptoms
> - The Six Tissue States of the Ancient Greeks and Eclectic Doctors – finding the root of the imbalance
> - A plant's action according to taste and chemistry
> - Personality of the person and how they deal with stress, both difficult and happy
> - How the plant moves energy from inside the body to outside, from the head to the feet and vice versa
> - How plants affect the spirit and soul body as energy moves through the auric field and into an individual's nervous system
> - Organ systems – deficiency and excess
> - Plants that are adaptogenic and effect hormonal firings

Simples and Formulas

These two seemingly opposing philosophies are only one of the great debates on how to practice herbalism. I don't take a hard line on either of them, for both methods have value and work.

Simple defines the art of recommending one plant to be used at one time per person. This method is especially useful in complex cases, because it gives a practitioner the ability to gauge where and how the plant will move energy and how a person might react to that movement. I also enjoy working this way when a client is taking numerous medications. Sometimes, one plant is all that is needed.

To use a *formula* is to employ two or more plants at a time. Many believe that a formula capitalizes on the synergy (harmonious alliance) between plants. They believe that this matrix has a multidimensional effect on illness. It is useful when the symptom picture is diverse and complex. I commonly use no more than 2-4 plants in a formula. Once in a blue moon, I'll emulate a historical

Chinese formula that uses 13 plants for a client, but again, that is rare.

Many will argue that the simples method allows a person's spirit to more effectively meet and work with a plant's spirit. That is true, but I believe that also occurs when a formula is used. When herbalism is practiced well, the bond between person and plant is powerful and will not be diminished because a simple or a formula is used.

In all cases, I believe that, besides the clinical effects herbs have on the body, the vibration of simple or formula sounds a note or chord that moves the dissonance of illness and unrest in the body. This sound helps retrain function and restore balance in the body, supporting and creating a terrain that illness and unrest cannot thrive in. This is the goal of alternative medicine.

Energetic Terms

The term energetics has two meanings in plant medicines. It can be a class of plants that are warm and stimulating in nature, and are pungent and aromatic in taste. Or it can be the terms used to describe what a plant's action is in the body. Examples of energetic terms are anti-inflammatory, diaphoretic, anti-bacterial, carminative, etc.

A successful practice and understanding of plant medicines must include knowledge of this applied terminology. It makes it easier to understanding what plants do, and easier to read and understanding good resources about them.

A basic list of energetics most useful to understanding applications can be found in Section 2 of this book.

Classification of Plant Medicines

A plant is classified, and its uses are defined in a variety of ways. While not everyone feels classification is beneficial, I find it can be, especially when first learning plant medicine.

Creating categories helps us efficiently organize information so that we can learn about plants, understand their relationships, differences, and uses both factually and historically. It is not, however, the only way we study and use plants.

Ways that we can categorize plants:

> ➢ By their botanical plant family
> ➢ By their taste and chemistry
> ➢ By their organ system affinity (what organs they act on)
> ➢ By their energetics (the action a plant has on the body or on illness)
> ➢ Whether they are stimulating or relaxing
> ➢ Which of the four qualities they possess – hot, cold, dry, and wet
> ➢ What illness they are used for
> ➢ Whether the plant is a tonic, medicine, or poison

Note: In the *Materia medica* chapter, I will write about each plant individually. Each of the above mentioned plant facts will be addressed. You will see most of these things listed.

The three terms we use in Western herbalism to classify plants are tonic, medicine, and poison. These help us determine why we might choose one plant over another, and understand the broader effects a plant may have on the body.

Tonic or food herbs nourish and tone the body over time. Dandelion root and leaf, burdock root, nettle leaf, seed and root, hawthorn, and raspberry leaf are a few that fall into this category. Tonics are thought to have stronger medicinal effects when used in formulas and in higher doses. I have seen great things happen in small doses and using them as simples, too. Tonics nourish and set the body up for positive long-term change.

Medicine herbs are used for acute illness and taken with care for a designated period of time, for they may cause imbalance when used inappropriately. Examples of herbs as medicines are ephedra, licorice root, goldenseal, marshmallow root, valerian, uva ursi, and blue cohosh. There are times when a medicine herb may be used as a tonic, but that concept is for more advanced work.

Poisons are plants that may be used in tiny doses, and only under the supervision of someone trained in their application. They can elicit a strong reaction when used improperly, such as vomiting and even death. When taken in their proper dose, they are excellent support. I feel that everyone should learn to use a poison early in their practice, because they can! Poke root, pullsatilla, lobelia, and may apple are examples of this class of herbs. The two we will discuss in this book are poke root and lobelia.

The Ever Important Herbal Tonic

Herbal tonics are a class of plant medicine that nourishes, tones, and retrains the body. Their effects can be felt immediately, depending on dosage, plant, and person. But the best results are seen when ingested over a long period of time. They work slowly to inspire deep and long standing internal changes.

Tonics can be taken as teas, tinctures, or eaten as food. And dosages vary. I prefer to use small doses, especially if using tonics for non-disease deficiency. For example, I may recommend a client take 5-10 drops of the nervine blue vervain 3-4 times daily for 6-12 months. When they first begin, the change in feeling and mood may be subtle. After a week, however, muscles may feel more relaxed, and mood may be more flexible. With each passing day, more improvements will be seen.

That is the work of tonics. As stated, they slowly and surely retrain internal patterns, which eventually become more consciously noted by our mind and body. How do plants do this? By coaxing organ systems and tissue to remember balance and function by either stimulating or relaxing, and through one or more of the following qualities: moistening to soften, drying to harden, heating to disperse energy, and cooling to restrain it.

There are tonics for all the organ systems and body functions. We have liver, urinary tract, immune, nervous system, digestive, heart, adrenal, and lymphatic tonics. These are all important for achieving optimal health. In true Western herbalism, balance is the key to health and prevention.

An herbalist assesses imbalanced organ systems, theorizes on the root of the problem, takes into account how long that imbalance has been in cycle, and recommends the most appropriate plant or combination of plants to refocus energy and function. A client can expect to follow a tonic protocol with some variation depending on how quickly the body responds.

Note: In the event that disease has already taken root and become a part of the organic nature of the individual, or a drug has affected the natural tendency of the person, tonics are less effective. While many herbs and tonics have great effects on disease, the intention and approach will differ slightly, depending on the person and the illness. Remember, it is illegal to treat disease or prescribe. We recommend and work with system imbalances and organ system function/energetics.

The Four Qualities and Two Tensions - Hot, Cold, Dry, Wet, Stimulating, and Relaxing

The four qualities and two tensions are words we use in herbalism to describe the effect a plant has on the body, both inside and out. They are also terms we use to describe the personality of a person and their condition. Each quality and tension embodies and describes how energy is moving and functioning.

The application of these terms have been used in various ways in the ancient traditions of the Chinese, in Ayurvedic medicine, and the Tissue State practice of the Ancient Greeks. They are also used in the younger system of Western herbalism.

Stimulating and relaxing define the initial effect a plant has on the body. One may use a plant to stimulate or relax any function of the body or organ system. For instance, blue vervain and motherwort relax the nervous system and muscles, while ginger and garlic stimulate the blood, immune system, and other organs.

The interesting and more complex aspect of this is what occurs after the initial relaxing or stimulating. These effects are a topic for a more advanced book, but one that I will begin to address now using the plants mentioned above to illustrate this new point. When one relieves the nervous system of tension, as we may do with blue vervain or motherwort, circulation is improved, and therefore slightly stimulated. The plants that stimulate also elicit an opposite reaction. When we use warming plants, such as garlic or ginger, to relieve internal cold that causes tension amongst other imbalances, we inspire a person to relax. More on this will be found under the descriptions for hot, cold, dry, and wet.

Hot, cold, dry, and wet are polar opposites, just as stimulating and relaxing. When we begin to study them, we study each individually so that we can best understand their characteristics. Let's look at how the warming ginger illustrates the quality hot.

Let's say you have a cold. For your remedy, you choose a simple few cups a day of warm and stimulating ginger tea with honey. The ginger will warm the blood and stimulate immunity to help the body fight infection. As it does so, it will act as a diaphoretic (fever reducer) to help manage the low-grade fever you may also have. It will also help thin, dry, and expectorate mucous in the sinuses and/or chest and act as a mild anti-spasmodic to assist cough management. Are you prone to colds turning into more complex infections, such as bronchitis or pneumonia? Combine it with something that further potentiates immunity and protects the lungs, such as licorice or elecampane with calendula or echinacea.

In this scenario, the ginger moved energy by heating and stimulating. But it did more than move with heat. What did it move? Coldness. It also thinned to slightly dry up mucous. The four qualities interact and move together. One cannot shift without the others shifting, nor can one exist without the other. They are interconnected, just as yin and yang are.

There are many ways to explain the four qualities and their complexities. I choose to explain them as they relate to the practice of the Ancient Greeks, for that is one of the traditions that Western herbalism is based on. You'll find basic descriptions below. They are oversimplified for the beginning herbalist.

Learning tip: As you read about each, taste a plant that represents the quality. Examples are included.

Hot

The Light Side of Heat

Heat can melt wax, thin oil, and evaporate fluids. It is the sun that inspires plants to grow, and the element that makes us want to live out our dreams.

Heat stimulates internal function. It has effects on all systems of the body, from the liver, the heart and circulatory system, to immunity, fight or flight, and digestion and cellular metabolism.

Just as heat affects wax, oil, and water in the environment, it also warms to thin and separate fluids in our body, such as blood that is cold and thick or mucous that is stuck, causing congestion. This improves blood flow, how hormonally coded messages travel, how nutrients move to their respective cells, how those cells purge waste for elimination, and how said waste is passed to organs of elimination.

When your immune system is under-functioning, if you feel constantly cold, or feel digestion is weak, we herbalists may use a tonic plant that is warming to stimulate function.

The Dark Side of Heat

With all the good that heat does, though, when in excess, it can worsen health. It may exacerbate inflammatory conditions, become a driving force in autoimmune diseases, be a part of an over ambitious immune system causing a high fever with an acute illness, or be the cause of excessive hot blood and an easily angered person. In short, too much heat leads to physical and emotional breakdown due to over combustion. When left unchecked, heat becomes destructive.

Taste

We'll talk about applying warming plants or acute illness and first aid in Section 2. For now, taste a plant. It will give you an idea of what warming plants do. Chew on some cardamom seeds, nibble a bit of fresh ginger root or dried licorice root, have a cup of nettle leaf tea. Plants that are warming are composed of the following tastes: pungent, aromatic bitters, and sometimes salty.

Tip: Not all plants that warm are drying. Some are moistening due to their high resin content, a detail that will be addressed in the *Materia medica*.

Hot Fact: Warm things don't just excite folk and function. People react differently to heating plants, depending on their disposition. Some people taste a warming plant and cold is moved. Some may feel simulated, while others feel relaxed. Some students and clients have told me that they can even feel cold expel through their mouth upon chewing a cardamom seed. Note your reaction!

Cold

<u>The Light Side of Cold</u>

Cold freezes fluid and hardens fat. It imparts a stillness that is
necessary to process and organize, allowing us to bring order to
function. Whether it is resting to digest food, process
information, or sleeping to heal, cool is the calmness necessary
to achieve these goals.

Cold in tissue constricts to bind and make solid, which helps
tissue and cells hold their tone. It also keeps heat to functional
levels so that it doesn't cause tissue to breakdown from calidity,
the blood to boil, or the nervous and immune systems to become
over excited.

<u>The Dark Side of Cold</u>

Excessive cold, however, can cause depression in endocrine and
immune function. It congeals blood, making it too thick, which
may cause circulatory and heart problems. As circulatory power
is reduced, our immune system is further weakened, nutrition
traveling to cells is slowed, and hormonally coded messages are
less effectively sent through the blood.

Emotional depression is also caused by cold. As rigidity of the
body, mind, spirit, and soul set in, we may retreat into our selves
and disengaging from our life in a community. This denies our
soul its work and purpose, further perpetuating depression.

<u>Taste</u>

Nibble a dandelion root, drink a cup of dandelion leaf tea, taste
goldenseal or gentian root tincture, eat a raspberry, or a
cranberry raw and unsweetened! Plants that are cooling come in
different flavors - sours, cold stimulating bitters, acrid bitters,
and sometimes salty.

Cold Fact: Cold stimulating bitters like dandelion root don't simply
cool. Cool bitters stimulate to excite stagnant function that is
allowing heat to build in tissue and blood, stimulating an organ
system to remember how to do its job. This mobilizes heat that is
stuck into action, thereby cooling. This breaks the tension that
builds from stuck (stagnant) function and can make some people

feel relaxed. Sours, such as raspberry leaf and hawthorn, cool blood, calm function, and astringe and balance tissue and muscle tone. They literally expunge heat that is acting irrationally and in disproportion to what is necessary for function. They also assist cell repair post cooling, facilitating efficient organ system and tissue function.

Dry

The Light Side of Dry

Just as with cold and hot, dry and moist are a part of a matrix that maintains and is essential to health. The two balance each other in tissue, blood, and function.

Dryness creates a tension in tissues and cells to help them remain stable and hold their tone. It provides protection, forbidding particles that should be kept out from penetrating the wall of the tissue or cell, and keeping in that which should be contained.

The Dark Side of Dry

In excess, however, dryness will cause tissue and mucous to harden, blood to lack nutrition, and oil, water, and digestive function to be impaired. As a result, foods will not be broken down properly in the stomach or absorbed in the small intestine. This puts stress on the colon and other organs of elimination. Excess dry will also prevent the blood from interfacing properly with cells that need to receive nutrition and purge waste, for it will be too low in electrolytes, oil, and water. That goes without mentioning its affect on mucous membranes that will be irritated and dry.

Taste

Dry plants of a cool and astringent nature are yellow dock root, a cup of raspberry leaf tea, and dandelion leaf.

Dry plants that are pungent aromatics (warm nature) are cardamom seeds, ginger, and sage leaf tea, which brings up oil and helps with fat digestion, but dries water.

Dry Tip: Sometimes a person will have very dry skin or constipation but have a wet runny nose or wet cough. That's the body's attempt to balance dryness. Instead of drying that one wet symptom, I often have people moisten the dry symptom. After a few weeks of this, wet and dry balance, with both symptoms being relieved. Plants to try are fenugreek, plantain leaf, marshmallow root, or garlic.

Wet

The Light Side of Water

Water is vital support for tissues and cells. It provides a different sort of protective element than dryness, for it dilutes and carries away toxins that may be damaging. Water is nourishment that helps deepen our emotional and physical health in otherwise unachievable ways.

Internally and externally, water in our cells and tissues help us maintain a balanced state of calmness, permeability, and flexibility. It soothes and relieves irritation that comes with heat, dryness, and hardness.

Water in combination with other elements in the blood is a nutrient transportation and waste management system. Balanced with the appropriate minerals, electrolytes, and fats, water thins and moves blood to carry nutrition to cells, assists nutrient absorption, and stimulates cells to purge waste. It then helps deliver waste to the proper eliminatory organ for excretion.

The Dark Side of Water

Excess water can cause thin and cold blood that lacks nutrition or fats. With the lack of heat, circulatory and muscular weakness and breakdown can occur. Think of a water balloon that sits too long. The water eventually breaks down the rubber, and it bursts. The same thing can happen in the circulatory system, as blood vessels breakdown and rupture. Hemorrhoids are one example of this.

Too much water can also cause stagnation. If organs of elimination (colon, kidney, bladder, lungs, skin) aren't working well, waste and water build in the cells. In this case, instead of cooling, the stagnant fluid creates heat. Opening organs of elimination with cool stimulating bitters can help relieve this problem.

There is also an emotional backlash to excess water. In some cases, too much water causes us to drown in our own sea of over emotion.

<u>Taste</u>

For salty plants that moisten, try burdock root and nettle leaf tea.

For sweet plants that moisten, try marshmallow root tea and milky oat tincture.

The Spectrum of Taste; Going Back to Plant Medicine Roots

In days past, the internal plant-to-person relationship began with taste. Taste doctors would decide a plant's ability to cool, heat, dry, moisten, calm, or stimulate. They would appraise the plants basic actions, determine specific medicinal uses, and assess which organs each plant had an affinity for. Their theories would then be applied to patients, at which time they would take notes and observe the degree of success or failure. Taste paved the road to recovery.

Today, many modern herbalists are recalling this old medical habit to move clients to better health and balance. From history and through experience, we know that when a plant in its purest taste touches the tongue, a chemical reaction inspires a multitude of energetic responses that are felt throughout the body. We match the taste to a person after deciding tissue state, organ system imbalances, symptom picture, and malady and/or complaint. A single plant or formula is recommended in the hope that our client may achieve their healing goals. Goals may include improving digestion, curbing sugar cravings, balancing anxiety, or fighting infection.

There are six basic tastes in herbalism, some of which I spoke about in the section on hot, dry, cold, and wet. They are cooling bitter, acrid bitter, warming aromatic bitter/pungent, sour, sweet, and salty. Each plant within these categories wields its own flavorful variation, together creating a taste spectrum. For example, gentian root is extremely bitter, but it is also a kin through flavor to the less bitter, slightly sweet, and salty dandelion root. Yet despite their taste differences, both roots are valid cooling bitters.

In the example, dandelion root demonstrates another point to consider when studying taste. It bears a different complexity in its flavor then gentian root by embodying three flavors – cooling bitter, slightly sweet, and salty. This is not unusual. In fact, it is closer to the norm. Most plants have more than one taste. And each one, whether perceived by the user or not, adds to the plant's medicinal attributes.

There is much we can learn from this perspective on taste. Three are important to remember now.

1. We learn how plants are similar and different in their actions and personalities.
2. We understand that a plant has many amazing attributes that are defined through the language of energetics (i.e. diuretic, carminative, cholagogue, etc.). This manner of understanding plant medicines is important now, because Western marketing teaches that a plant has one use which is malady specific. For example, western marketing tells us that echinacea is for cold and flu and St. John's wort is for depression. It is time to unlearn this, for it is not how herbs work.
3. Taste instructs us on the balance and true nature of the plant as a healer. It finely illustrates how plants inspire our body to do their job by way of the following qualities: heating, cooling, moistening, drying, relaxing, and stimulating. A foundation that we will explore throughout this book, using first aid and acute infections of the respiratory tract to illustrate.

I will not delve too deep into the function of each taste in this book. But for now, it's good to be aware of the tastes through the four qualities (hot, cold, dry, wet), and the two tensions (stimulating and relaxing).

Taste Exercises

We all perceive taste in our own way, just like scent. To broaden one's perspective on the essence of a flavor is fun and educational. Set tasting sessions with groups of friends and others interested in studying herbal medicine, or just with your housemates. Taste a plant and talk about where the taste moves in the body, what you feel on your tongue, and the way it makes you feel.

Word to the wise: There are many poisonous plants, some which look similar to innocuous ones. Please know or have someone who knows the plant you are about to ingest before going on a plant tasting binge in the wild.

Chapter 2

Aromatics as Medicines and Aromatherapy

Aromatic medicines have been around for thousands of years, with the modern version of aromatherapy being in existence for nearly 100 years. Despite this, it's still a misunderstood and controversial healing art. And why shouldn't it be? Commercial products claim "aromatherapy" while they employ chemical scents that are not medicinal, and natural product companies overuse natural scents. We are inundated and overwhelmed with pointless and senseless scent. It has become the anti-medicine.

There is a way to reclaim aromatics as a viable healing art. As consumers, we can separate the baseless from the functional. I achieve that with my clients and students by asking them to eliminate scent from daily use (scented soaps, detergents, hair and body products, perfumes, etc.). Then, I recommend they choose the scents they want in the products they want. The caveat is that what they pick must be natural (not synthetic), and serve a specific purpose. For example, if they need rose water for their skin or would like an essential oil salt bath that treats a specific ailment, then that is what they choose.

With this, people become educated and aware of what and why they use a scent. They simplify their lives and make conscious and deliberate decisions about what they put on their bodies.

What is Aromatherapy?

Aromatherapy is the external application and inhalation of aromatic plants as medicines. Here are a few ways we can do this.

- ➢ Adding essential oils to salves, liniments, bath products, or other products for topical application
- ➢ Using fresh plants to make wreaths or herb bundles to hang in homes
- ➢ Working with fresh plants with our hands to emit scent
- ➢ Cooking with herbs that scent the home with vapors
- ➢ Burning plants
- ➢ The use of aromatic teas for steam inhalation or bathing

Why and How Does Aromatherapy Work?

When used with specific intent, aromatics and essential oils have profound effects on our psyche, quickly changing how we feel about a situation at hand, or, when used regularly, undoing the cumulative effects that stress has on our body.

Let's say that a general ill feeling comes over you in response to a stressful event. If our body's memory serves us right, it is a familiar feeling, for we often react the same way to stress. But we have an aromatherapy formula with us, and we take a moment to inhale its scent. When we smell, hormonally coded messages are sent from the brain to corresponding systems. It is a process that takes place in less than a second. Depending on what we smell, we can excite or relax the nervous system and brain to affect mood, positively changing our mind's perception of the event at hand and how we feel about it.

With the regular use of therapeutic scent, we have the ability to move beyond merely changing how we feel in an instant to retraining our body's reaction emotionally, physically, and chemically, to stressful situations. In the end, our ability to adapt to stress, in both our sensory and emotional bodies, will have a beneficial effect on our physical healing.

Retraining is the key word here. Chronic disease and disorders that affect our physical and emotional health worsen with stress. When we change our perspective and reaction to stress, we then affect the physical patterns that drive disease and ill health. Our health improves and becomes more sustainably functional.

Stress relief can also encourage a positive outlook, one that inspires faith and trust, and increases personal insight. While these effects are not in direct relation to what needs healing, our new frame of reference supports a larger and more permanent healing process.

What is Aromatherapy Good For?

Aromatics can:

- Promote general health and well being
- Reduce stress or depression
- Sedate or invigorate

- Stimulate sensory awareness
- Boost immune function
- Relieve sinus congestion or a spastic cough
- Provide muscular pain relief
- Relieve emotional pain associated with physical pain

Aromatherapy works well for:

- Nervous system imbalances
- Insomnia
- Depressed immunity
- Hormonal imbalances
- Autoimmune diseases
- Memory, by stimulating parts of the brain
- Used as aphrodisiacs
- Spiritual and soul healing

Why I Love Using Essential Oils

As an herbalist and aromatherapist, I use aromatics in my practice regularly – at home, in classes, and with clients. Here are a few great reasons for doing so.

> ➤ They potentiate salves, making them more powerful and versatile. I can increase the anti-bacterial, anti-inflammatory, and anti-spasmodic effects with essential oils. The addition of scent to salves also capitalizes on another therapy. When things have a pleasing scent, people are more likely to use them. Chronic and acute physical pain can drive emotional pain, which, in turn, worsens physical pain. Both the physical and emotional pain is made more bearable and greatly decreased with scent.
> ➤ Using essential oils as a therapy instead of plants internally can help avoid drug-herb interactions or simply lessen what a client has to take internally.
> ➤ Aromatherapy can be the gateway therapy for alternative medicine. Back in the herb store days, and still now, I get clients that don't want to take plants internally. They don't trust it or are afraid. Using external medicines that are beneficial is an excellent medium for them. They feel relief, and it builds their trust in plants. Sometimes, this makes them more open to internal remedies.

How Aromatherapy Came to Be

In 1928, a Frenchman by the name of Rene-Maurice Gattefosse was working at his family's lavender distillery when his arm was badly burned. In his haste, he submerged his arm in a vat of lavender pure essential oil. To his surprise, the pain quickly dissipated. He also noticed that his arm healed quickly with no scaring or infection.

The union of lavender and Gattefosse sparked a revitalization of a healing art that was thousands of years old and had been lost for nearly 40 years. In the late 1800's, aromatics were downgraded from their historically medicinal status to being typecast as for perfumery only.

Lavender inspired Gattefosse to re-invent the field of aroma-medicines as "aromatherapy," a term he coined in the book he published in 1937 titled, *Gattefosse's Aromatherapy*. It was the first of its kind.

The Practice of Aromatherapy is another notable work that was written in the 1960's by Dr. Jean Valnet. The book is a documentation of Dr. Valnet's work using essential oils to heal the wounds of soldiers in the war, and later as medicine to help soldiers heal from Post Traumatic Stress Disorder associated with emotional distress.

Another historic contribution to the field of aromatherapy was published in 1977 and written by Robert Tisserand. It is a lovely work titled, *The Art of Aromatherapy*. His book inspired the practice of aromatherapy in America. While each of the above books is an important reference and study of the practice of aromatherapy, I find Tisserand's work to be especially so, because he documents much of the historical practice of using aromatics as medicines for the healing of the mind, and physical, emotional, and spiritual body.

Basics of Essential Oil Formulation

What is an Essential Oil?

An essential oil is a liquid that is the result of the distillation of plant matter. The liquid is called oil, but it is not a fatty substance. An essential oil is a volatile plant essence that is subject to evaporation and sensitive to heat and light.

Parts of the plant that may be used are the bark, resin, leaves, twigs, flowers, grass, and fruit.

What are Carrier Oils, and How do You Use Them?

A carrier oil is a fatty oil, such as sweet almond oil or grape seed oil. To dilute essential oils, you add them to a carrier oil. There are several reasons for doing this.

1. One needs medium to dilute the essential oils in, for they are caustic to the skin when used undiluted (neat). While it is appropriate to use some essential oils undiluted on minor burns, bug bites, or pimples, it is not recommended otherwise.
2. Carrier oils allow for the essential oils to be evenly distributed across the desired area. This is impossible to do without a carrier oil, for the molecular structure and consistency of an essential oil is so small that it will stay in the spot it is applied. A salve can also be used for this purpose.
3. An essential oil is properly absorbed when a carrier oil is used. In fact, a carrier oil serves much the same purpose alcohol, honey, and vinegar do in internal plant preparations. The essential oil with the carrier passes easily into the fluid surrounding the cells beneath the skins surface, into the lymph ducts and capillaries, and into the bloodstream to circulate throughout the body via fluid transport.

There are many different kinds of carrier oils, from apricot oil to jojoba oil. I keep at least three on hand in my practice, and I use them according to the person's skin type, their condition, and the season and climate. Here is the short list of oils I recommend.

> ➤ Normal skin: apricot oil and jojoba oil
> ➤ Dry/sensitive skin: avocado oil, apricot oil, almond oil, and aloe vera oil
> ➤ Oily skin: jojoba oil
> ➤ Mature/aging skin: avocado oil and almond oil

Dilutions of Essential Oils to Carrier Oils

When we add the formula of essential oils we have chosen to the carrier oil, we chose the reason for making the product and follow dilution guidelines. Here are a few dilution basics.

> ➤ Massage, bath, and body oils: ½-1% dilution (3-6 drops of essential oil per ounce of carrier oil). Less is more here, especially in those with sensitive skin and autoimmune disorders.
> ➤ Inhalation: 1-2 drops in a bowl containing 2 cups of hot water or on a tissue for relief of sinus problems or emotional distress.
> ➤ Muscle tension or strain: 2-5% dilution (12-30 drops per 1 ounce of carrier oil or salve) for application to affected area. This would not be used a for full body application.
> ➤ For perfumery and meditation: ½-1% dilution (3-6 drops per 1 ounce of carrier oil).

If formulating for the elderly or children aged 5-12, use the ½% dilution. If you are making products for infants to four year olds, use 1-2 drops per ounce of carrier oil.

The Importance of Scent in Formulation

A person's experience with scent is subjective and unique. What we believe smells wonderful may smell offensive to others. It is therefore important to take personal preference into account, because the therapy will be lost if an adverse emotional reaction is elicited.

I have also found that while someone may dislike the scent of an oil on its own, they sometimes don't mind it in a formula. Also, one's perception of a scent can change, for hormones in the body can affect our perception of scent. Times we may dislike something are during pregnancy, cancer treatments, stressful times, menstruation, or acute illness.

Formulation for Acute Infection

When using an aromatherapy formula for relief of an acute illness, I recommend simple formulas used for a specific period of time. For instance, if using essential oils for a virus or bacterial infection, I would suggest that the formula be employed for 10-14 days. If treating a fungal infection that is topical, I would use the formula until five days after the infection in completely cleared.

Here are some basic guidelines for choosing your essential oils.

> Know your symptom picture and choose oils accordingly. Keep your formula simple to make a powerful healing agent that saves resources and cuts costs, especially when beginning your practice. Generally, formulas for acute illnesses only need 2-3 essential oils.

> Include one oil that is an effective immune booster. Unbeknownst to many, adding one from this category makes a world of difference. It can often mean the difference between getting full blown sick and being a bit under the weather.

> Nervine or sedative. Include an oil that supports relaxation. When we rest, we heal. Oils that are calming also have anti-microbial effects.

> Specifics to infection. If you can, employ an essential oil that is an anti-infective agent and is specific to what you believe you may have or have been diagnosed with. In other words, if you have been diagnosed with strep throat, choose thyme or cinnamon, for they are especially effective against the bacteria. For more information on this, check the *Materia medica.*

Choosing Essential Oils for Bath

When choosing essential oils for the bath, it is best to use caution. Stick with oils that aren't irritating, such as flowers, resins, some trees, and some herbs.

Tip: If you have very sensitive skin, be sure to do a skin test before using essential oils in your tub. Take one drop of an essential oil you plan to use in the tub and add it to a teaspoon of carrier oil. Apply it to a place on your body that tends to be more sensitive or rash up. For some it's the back, for others it's the arms or a small unnoticeable place on the face or neck. If there is no irritation, then the oil is safe for bath use.

Warning: Essential oils that should never be used in baths are: mints, camphor, wintergreen, cinnamon, ginger, black pepper, and most citrus oils. They could/will irritate the skin.

Oils to use in small amounts are: clove, cardamom, rosemary, eucalyptus (use only a few drops per bath), grapefruit (unless sensitive skin).

What to do if you take a bath in something that gives you a rash.

1. Get out of the tub and rub your whole body down with unscented lotion or olive oil. (I prefer olive oil but have used unscented lotion in a pinch.)
2. Take a cold wet bath towel and begin gently applying it to the affected areas.
3. Continue applying oil or lotion and the wet towel until the itching begins to feel better, and the redness is lessened. This process can take about 10-15 minutes.

Supply List for Formulating

You will need:

- Labels. Label everything you make and date it.
- Carrier oil(s) of choice. I generally use a 50/50 mix of almond oil and jojoba oil.
- Essential oils.
- Bottles for mixing in. You may choose ½, 1, 2, or 4 ounce sizes. Glass amber brown or cobalt blue bottles are best. Colored bottles protect the integrity of the product from light. But, in a pinch, I have also used Franks Hot Sauce bottles, maple syrup bottles, and mason jars. All are clear glass, but if the formulas are used quickly and are kept out of the sun, it is fine. If purchasing bottles, avoid the ones with droppers. The oil travels up the glass dropper and into the rubber part, eating it away and contaminating the oil formula with rubber - YUCK. You need bottles with lids.

Making the Formula

Choose your essential oils, then mix them with the carrier oil in the bottle. Be sure to follow the proper dilutions (number of essential oil drops you add per ounce of carrier oil).

Drop by drop you will make your formula. Remember, you cannot subtract a drop. Smell the oils chosen and decide which you would like more of. It is important to learn which are very strong. Some, such as lavender and rose, will take over the formula, depending on what you mix them with. I recommend adding equal drops of each, say one drop of each, shaking, smelling, then deciding which you would like to add more of.

Be sure to stay within the boundaries of dilution. And remember, it takes 24 hours for the formula to meld. The scent of the formula will continue to change for about a week. But the general scent will immerge in 24 hours.

Write everything you put in the bottle on your label and date it. If you feel so inclined, name your formula or simply write it's uses on the label.

Your oil formula will be good for 4-6 weeks. If you use 20% jojoba oil, however, it will last indefinitely.

Tip: To preserve and extend the shelf life of your carrier oil formulas, salves, and creams naturally, add 20% jojoba oil to your products. Jojoba oil has an oily consistency but is a wax. It has the same molecular structure as sebum produced by the skin. It doesn't clog pores, and won't go rancid.

Chapter 3

Extracting the Medicine;

Making Alcohol Tinctures and Infused Oils

When we make plant medicines, we wield the power of a centuries-old practice with the intent to incite positive change. As we work our hands to prepare the plants for extraction, our pace and mind slow. We step back in time to a place where there were no machines to make the work go faster and where computers didn't exist. The only distractions might have been an accidental spill, a child crying, or a neighbor knocking.

Making medicines the old way in this new age strengthens our focus, will, and discipline, for those are the tools called on to do the task. This presents a challenge for some, because many of us are not used to using our hands and minds this way.

Each person I have taught medicine-making to goes through their own process. Some prepare things with confidence and grace, enjoying every moment. Others question every move they make or judge themselves harshly for mistakes. Regardless, the work becomes easier as you attune yourself to the feel of the plant in your hands and to the process. With the remedies successfully made and eventually applied, your confidence and self-esteem will grow. This will make you a strong and proficient herbalist.

Medicine Making - An Herbalist's Menstruums

Medicine making is not difficult. If you can follow directions and measure, you can do it. There are some things to have an understanding of first, though. If you're taking time and using resources to make the medicines, then you want to do it well.

What is a menstruum, and which are used in plant medicine?

A menstruum is the fluid solvent used to extract the chemical constituents from plants that we use as therapy. In this book, we will focus on using alcohol, water, and oil. The most common menstruums are:

- Alcohol of high quality and high alcohol content (95% +)
- Vegetable Glycerin
- Water
- Vinegar
- Honey
- Oil

What plants should be extracted in what menstruums?

Most people believe that if you can make a water infusion with a plant, you can make a tincture or vice versa. Unfortunately, that's not the case. Some chemical constituents are soluble in alcohol and oil, while others are soluble in water and honey. Nutrients are soluble in water, honey, and vinegar. It's important to know what you need to make the most effective medicines. You'll find this information in the *Materia medica*.

Because this is a beginning herb book, I won't be going into great detail about the chemistry behind medicine making. If you're interested in that, you will find books on the subject of plant chemistry in the Bibliography.

What part of the plant should be used, and should it be used fresh or dried?

It's important to know which part of the plant holds the medicine and, if multiple parts are medicinal, how to process each and what it's used for. Some plants must be used fresh, some can be used both fresh or dried, while others need to be dried or cured for months. You will see this information in the *Materia medica* as well.

What is the best menstruum-to-plant dilution for a potent medicine?

Tinctures that are properly labeled will be marked with the dilution. For example, you will see 1:1, 1:2, 1:3, or 1:5, to name a few. The first number denotes the ratio of plant used by weight. The second number is the amount of fluid by volume. If it is a 1:2 dilution, there was 1 part plant used per 2 parts menstruum. This will be addressed further in tincture making and in the *Materia medica*.

What is the shelf life of the product?

This varies and will be addressed per product and in each process.

What is a basic dose, and what are the applicable uses of each plant?

Again, this varies per person, per malady, and per plant. Information on dosage and use will be found in Sections 2 and 3 of this book.

The Menstruums - Oil and Alcohol

Oil

Fatty substances have been used to extract plant medicines for thousands of years. Proof is seen in the papyrus drawings of Ancient Egypt, which depict Egyptians doing various things while wearing what are called *ungent cones* on their heads. The cone was shaped from solid fats that flowers, resins, roots, and barks were macerated in. The ungent cone would melt slowly in the day's heat, releasing the extracted scent, and melting the fat to drip down the head.

These days, we use cold pressed vegetable or nut oils (most commonly, extra virgin olive oil) or jojoba oil (which is actually a liquid wax) for extraction. Sometimes they are solid, and sometimes they are liquid. The infused oils, as they are called, are used in salve making, lip balms, bath and body products, hand creams, ear oils, and products both medicinal and for perfumery.

While most infused oils tend to be employed for external use, there are some we use in cooking. They are fragrant and delicious, often containing herbaceous plants that are grown in kitchen gardens. Rosemary, thyme, oregano, and garlic are just a few favorites that folks like to use. They are a lovely addition to food preparation. Unless made by measuring, they are only marginally medicinal.

Alcohol

Alcohol is another menstruum that has forever been a part of medicine making. From the Ancient Egyptians and Medieval herbalists, who macerated plants and dried fruits in wine, to the Germans, who brewed clary sage and other beneficial botanicals into beers, history is full of many methods and perspectives involving the use of alcohol to make herbal remedies.

Alcohol is still widely used today, in home and commercial products alike, and will be one of your main menstruums. The plant part is placed in the alcohol to macerate (soften and break down), allowing the alcohol to draw out the chemical constituents used for medicine. This takes eight weeks or more. I, personally, allow roots to macerate for up to nine months. When ready, the plant is pressed out, leaving the alcohol infusion, which is called the tincture.

We modern herbalists can easily purchase high quality alcohol to make tinctures with. I'm picky about mine. I want it to be grain, yeast, and allergen free, because I work with a lot of clients who are sensitive to those things. Therefore, the product needs to be distilled from something besides grains and not be brandy or wine, which has yeast in it. I also want a high alcohol content to ensure maximum potency, and a shelf life of 10+ years with little to no chance of mold.

For this reason, I use, and recommend my students use, distilled organic grape or organic cane alcohol. They are both 190 proof (96% alcohol). That's a lot of alcohol, but it's necessary. Fresh plants have water in them by nature. So if you use an alcohol with a high water content, it often leads to mold and a far shorter shelf life. That wastes resources, time, and money. If you make your tincture properly, you'll have a long lasting, potent, and great product.

Over the years, I have softened my perspective on what alcohol can be used for making dry plant tinctures. Because the water is dehydrated out of the plant, and water needs to be added back in, I have written and promoted the use of potato vodka when working with dried plants.

I'd like to add a quick note on the cost of alcohol. Up front, it is expensive to purchase a gallon or ½ gallon of organic grape or cane alcohol. It can cost anywhere from $75-$140 per gallon, depending on how much you purchase at once. The cost is greatly decreased by going in with other herbalists and ordering in bulk.

When purchased by the gallon, however, your per ounce cost is between $ .56 and $1. Weigh that against paying $10 to $15 for a 1-ounce bottle of commercial tincture. The financial savings are notable, but so is the quality of product that you will have.

Making and Using Fresh and Dried Plant Tinctures

As mentioned above, a tincture is the product of a plant macerated in alcohol. It can be made with fresh or dried plant material. To take a tincture, you put your recommended number of drops (the dose) into a bit of water or juice. Some folks choose to use yogurt, smoothies, or applesauce.

I had a few students this year that had other ingenious ideas. One makes smoothies using fruit and herbs, pouring the mixture into ice cube trays. She pokes toothpicks in each one and freezes them. A cube is a serving. Her kids love them.

Another student discovered the art of making herb teas, and using them to make jello. Her herb of choice was holy basil. She adds grass fed beef gelatin and a bit of honey.

For people who have a difficult time taking tinctures made in alcohol, I recommend adding a tablespoon of hot water over the drops and allowing it to sit for a minute. Most of the alcohol will evaporate. I've found this to be an appropriate method for recovering alcoholics, those with alcohol allergies, and kids.

There are some that find this isn't enough. When this is the case, it is important to find another way to deliver the medicines. If the plant only extracts in alcohol, then find another plant that can be extracted in other ways.

While tinctures are typically for internal consumption, one can also use them externally. Some herbalists and medicine makers add tinctures to salves for specific reasons. For example, I might add a usnea tincture to a salve to strengthen the anti-bacterial and anti-fungal properties, or rosemary to stimulate circulation and infuse the salve with an anti-oxidant agent. You might also apply a tincture topically. I may drop yarrow tincture on a gaping wound to stop the bleeding, or St. John's wort tincture on that same wound to stop pain.

For the very sensitive, applying tinctures to the wrist to elicit a medicinal reaction is another common practice, and a great way to get a feel for the vibration of the plant if you're nervous about a drug interaction, or just plain nervous. Once you feel ready, you can begin taking the drop internally if you like.

Rules of Tincture Making

Our country is rich with philosophical variation on tincture making. My way is fairly simple, but does come with rules. Here are my top three tincture making rules.

1. Measure. A measured medicine yields measureable results. When we measure, we know the strength, can decide a dosage more easily, and understand the reaction. Tinctures that are measured properly and made with a high percentage alcohol also extract perfectly, are potent, and have a good long shelf life (10+ years).

2. As spoken about in the section on alcohol, know your alcohol content, and only use 190 proof with fresh plants. Fresh plants already have water in them. Adding more water causes excess oxidation, increases the risk of spoilage, and dilutes the extraction process, making for a less potent medicine.

    If it you are making a dried plant tincture, however, you can use a lower proof alcohol. I still prefer the 190 proof, because I want to have a flexible water to alcohol ratio. Fresh plants have different water contents, making the addition of water when making a dried plant tincture specific per plant.

    For example, Vodka is 60% alcohol and 40% water. Perhaps that ratio works for dried peppermint tincture. But the highly resinous dried calendula needs a higher percent of alcohol and lower of water. I want the flexibility to make those allowances. But you can get by using Vodka.

3. Know your plant-by-weight to menstruum-by-volume ratio. This information can be found in your *Materia medica*. Most fresh plant tinctures in this book will be 1:2 (that's 1 part plant by weight to 2 parts fluid by volume), while most dry plant tinctures will be 1:5.

Supplies for Making Fresh and Dried Plant Tinctures

*   Fresh and/or dried plant matter

- Filtered water (only if dried)
- High alcohol product (96%) or vodka (if fresh)
- Labels
- Something to press and stir with
- Canning funnel (optional)
- Measuring cup
- Mason jar of appropriate size
- Scale (While the awesome $150 scales are optimal, I have found digital kitchen scales from Target to work just fine. They run about $35 and are far more realistic for most people's budgets.)
- A dry, cool, dark place to store tinctures as they macerate

How to Make a Fresh Plant Tincture

1. Weigh your plant and figure your plant-to-fluid ratio. A fresh plant tincture is typically 1:2, meaning 1 part plant by weight to 2 parts fluid by volume. If you have 3 ounces of fresh yarrow, you will then need 6 ounces of high alcohol content fluid (organic grape, in this case).

2. Process your plant. That may mean chopping roots, cutting up flowers and leaves, and in some cases removing the plant's woody stems.

3. Put your plant in the jar and press it down, but not too tightly. We want the alcohol to fill in every little crack and crevice so as not to leave pockets of air, which can harbor mold and rot.

4. Pour the alcohol over the plant and be sure to mix it in well, than press it all down as far below the alcohol as possible. Be aware that with 1:2 fresh plant tinctures and some plants as 1:5 dried (such as calendula or yarrow) it is likely that the plant will rise above the alcohol as it absorbs the menstruum. You can re-press it as this occurs.

5. Shake the tincture. The advice of nearly all tincture makers is shake daily (or often as you remember) and let macerate for 6-8 weeks. I let my tinctures go longer, and I don't shake them as often. I like them to be calm and unruffled, but I like to agitate them and put some good human energy in, too.

Roots and seeds I let go for about half a year, all others about 2-3 months.

6. Label. The label should say the following:
   - The plant to alcohol ratio (example, 1:2)
   - Part of plant used
   - The Latin and common plant name
   - When and where it was harvested or purchased
   - The date you made the tincture

How to Make a Dried Plant Tincture

1. Weigh your plant and figure your plant-to-menstruum ratio. This is plant specific in many cases. For example, if you have 2 ounces of dried calendula flowers,1:5 is recommended. That is 1 part of plant by weight to 5 parts fluid by volume. 2 ounces of dried calendula x 5 parts fluid = 10 ounces! So we need 10 ounces of fluid.

2. Now that you know how much fluid you need, let's figure out how much alcohol to water you need. Yet another plant specific number. Let's stick with our calendula example. For calendula, of our 10 fluid ounces, we need 75% of that to be alcohol. Maddening to think about how many ounces of water and alcohol we need, isn't it? Especially if the ratio is 60/40 or 70/30. But it's really a simple equation.

   Let's do the alcohol. You multiply the number of total ounces of fluid (that's 10) by the % turned into a decimal number. In this case, 75% becomes .75. The equation looks like this: 10 x .75 = 7.5. So you need 7.5 ounces of alcohol. To figure your water is simply to subtract: 10 - 7.5 = 2.5. There you have it. It's quite simple.

   Remember, if you use vodka, you will not need to add water. It already has water in it.

3. Next you put your plant in the mason jar and add the room temperature water. Push the plant matter down in there the best you can. Let it sit for an hour or so in the water to reconstitute. If it is a root, I often let it sit overnight, covering the jar with a towel (leaving the lid on may cause mold). Not everyone does the reconstitution step. It feels somehow right

to me. I have also learned in the last couple of years that this is how the Alchemists do it.

If you are using vodka, you will not do this step.

4. Now that the herbs are reconstituted, add the alcohol. Use what you need to mix them in. I put the lid on and shake the jar. This is where chopsticks can come in handy. You can use them to get the air bubbles out. Afterward, press the plant down beneath the liquid with a potato masher. This feat is often easier with dried plant tinctures, because there is a higher fluid content added.

5. Shaking and maceration time. See step 5 above in Fresh Plant Tincture Making.

6. Now it's time to make the label. See step 6 above, but also add the percentage of alcohol (75%).

Making Infused Oils

Infused oils are most commonly used in the making of salves and creams. But you can also use them in bath salt products to add a bit of medicinal punch, or as a carrier oil for a specific purpose. For instance, I make a burn oil using St. John's wort infused oil with lavender and tea tree essential oils, and one for menstrual cramps with arnica infused oil as the base, with essential oils of lavender, ginger, and clary sage. It is applied directly over the uterus.

Remember when I said that formulating bath products isn't just about taking a bath and that it is also about getting an education? Infused oil formulation and salve making may be used the same way. When you are choosing what to use in your product, you need to know what plants do and how they affect the skin.

For information on plants used in infused oils and their applicable effects, refer to the *Materia medica* chapter on plants used in infused oils in Section 3. Plants included there are yarrow, arnica, chaparral, comfrey leaf, plantain leaf, calendula, and St. John's wort.

Steps for Making Dried Plant Infused Oils

1. Get a pint or quart sized wide mouth Mason jar. Sterilize it and make sure it's very dry. Size depends on how much oil you will make or what you have.

2. Weigh the plant material. You will need 5 ounces of oil per ounce of plant material. In other words, you will make a 1:5 dilution. (That translates into 1 part plant by weight to 5 parts fluid by volume.)

3. Add the plant material to the jar and pour the measured olive oil over it. Just as with tinctures, be sure to stir the oil to all parts of the jar. You don't want any air pockets. Press the plant material down as far as you can. To keep it down, you may need to do this daily as the plant becomes saturated and heavy.

   Tip: Mold and rancidity occur quickly. To protect my macerated oils from going bad, I always use a combination of 80% olive oil and 20% jojoba oil to macerate plants in. Jojoba oil has an oil consistency but is actually a wax distilled from a bean or seed. It doesn't go bad and will naturally prevent your products from mold rancidity. I also use a bit of high-grade alcohol in the process to assist extraction and prevent rancidity. Add about 1 ounce of 95% organic grape alcohol (not vodka because of the water) per pound of plant material.

4. Set in a warm place for 2-3 weeks. I don't use an outside heat source. You will notice that some people do. In the winter, I do set my oils by the heat vent.

5. When 2-3 weeks has passed, pour off the oil and press out through cheesecloth. Use your hands and get as much as you can.

6. Let your finished product sit overnight. If you see sludge on the bottom of the jar the next day, pour off the oil and discard the sludge. Store the oil in an airtight jar in a cool dry place. Colored glass is best, so I use amber brown bottles. Label and date everything! Include: the dilution (1:5 if a dried plant infusion), whether it was a fresh or dried

maceration, the date it was made (not just pressed), and what plants, oils and/or alcohol was used in the maceration process.

Steps for Making Fresh Plant Infused Oils

Weigh the plant material and put it in a large stainless steel bowl. For each pound of plant, add one ounce of alcohol. Stir the plant and alcohol, and then spread the plant out on a cookie sheet to wilt for 24 hours. This lessens the amount of water in your oil.

All other steps are the same as with dry plant material, except a few key points. The dilution of plant to oil will be 1:2, just as it is for fresh plant tinctures, not 1:5. Also, I recommend that people ALWAYS use alcohol and 20% jojoba oil to protect the integrity of your product when making fresh plant oils. Press the oil out in 2 weeks to avoid mold growth.

Storage, Shelf Life, and Labeling

Storage: I use amber brown bottles to store my macerated oils. Please keep them in a non-humid, heat and sunlight free place.

Shelf life: Oils that haven't been stabilized with alcohol and jojoba oil will have a shelf life of about 6-8 weeks. The fridge can prolong this by about a month, in some cases. Remember, use your nose and eyes. If it smells bad, it is. If it's got stuff growing on it, throw it out. Be sure to always check the smell of the oil before use. Mold and scum growth is a more likely problem in oils that were made with fresh plant material.

Label: Repeat from Chapter 2. Label everything! Write the following: date made and shelf life, all of the product's ingredients, product name and uses (if you're getting creative), instructions for use (especially if this is a gift), and the shelf life.

I highly recommend you keep notes on what you made, how you did it (especially if you deviate from special instructions), and what you put into it. Why? So you always know what you want to repeat, change, or experiments that failed.

Chapter 4

Making Salves and Lip Balms

Salve making is the heart of artful herbal medicine making. In my beginning herb class, the final project is a salve. Each student must formulate (figuring out what to use together and why), make the salve, and either write an advertisement about it or a paper on what it can be used for. It's fun, and most everyone gets into the process of creating their own product as they think about application and marketing. Some good folks even bring samples to share with classmates. And what they find is that salve making and formulation is a creative process, giving one a chance to expand on herbal ideas and bring that idea to fruition. It is powerful!

The first salve I made was a St. John's wort salve. After pressing the freshly infused oil, which is a gorgeous deep red, I set to work measuring, weighing, and heating. I had already decided that this salve would be simple, so I chose St. John's wort and calendula infused oils, with a few drops of lavender essential oil.

The salve was a beautiful red, and to this day is my favorite to make. I love that the little trio of plants (with the addition of a bit of jojoba oil as a preservative and beeswax to harden) does just about everything. It's our family's go-to salve!

I recommend you study the different infused oil plants in the *Materia medica*. You can even think of a few of your own. Now ask yourself, "What would my go-to salve be used for, and what would I need to put in it?"

Materials Lists

Ingredients

- Infused oils and carrier oils of choice. To preserve salves, I always add 15-20% jojoba oil to my recipe as a natural preservative. This will increase the shelf life of your product. Salves have a short shelf life of anywhere from six weeks to six months before they go rancid, depending on the environment they are kept in. Salves preserved with jojoba oil will keep indefinitely. This trick works for most all aromatherapy or oil based products and is a fact that I will repeat throughout this book.

- Beeswax.
- Essential oils of choice - Dilution of infused oils and carrier oils to essential oils in salve: A ½-1% dilution of carrier oil/salve base to essential oil is best for general purposes. That comes out to be about 3-6 drops of essential oil per ounce of salve. Therefore, if you are making 2 ounces of product, you would use 6-12 drops of essential oil total.

Tools

- Kitchen scale
- Double boiler (or Pyrex/stainless steel measuring cup with frying pan)
- Small glass containers to put your salve in
- Bamboo chopstick or small stainless steel spoon for mixing

Instructions for Making and For Use

1. To make the salve base, bring water to a boil in the double boiler and turn the heat down to a simmer. Add your carrier oil to receptacle or measuring cup that sits above or in the water.

2. Per cup of oil, and add 1 ounce of beeswax to the oil (using the scale to weigh). Let this simmer, stirring occasionally, until the beeswax is melted.

3. While you wait for the melting to occur, put the drops of essential oil into the glass jars that will hold the salve. When the base is finished, turn off the fire and allow it to cool while stirring for one minute. Do not let it harden. If it does, just turn on a low heat again until fully liquified.

4. Pour the melted salve into the jars with the essential oils, stir briefly, and then close the lids. Let the salves sit at room temperature until they harden.

5. Use as needed.

Storage Tips, Shelf Life, and Labeling

Storage Tips: Jars and containers for salves come in glass or plastic and in an array of sizes. It is nice to make them in 2 or 4 ounce sizes for the medicine cabinet. Smaller sizes, ¼-1 ounce, are nice for portable medicine bags. Keep out of sunlight and away from heat.

Shelf life: If you used jojoba oil, celebrate! Your salve is good for about a year. If you didn't, then watch the product. It may go rancid in 6-8 weeks. If you didn't make your infused oils the way I suggested, you'll get 6-8 weeks out of your salve as well.

Labeling: Date and label according to what was used in the product.

Sample Salve Formulas

Warming Foot Rub: jojoba oil, calendula infused oil; essential oils of cinnamon, clove, ginger, eucalyptus, sweet orange

Cooling Foot Rub: jojoba oil, yarrow infused oil; essential oils of lavender, peppermint, eucalyptus, vetiver

Muscle Madness Salve: St. John's wort, arnica infused oils; essential oils of eucalyptus, rosemary, peppermint, ginger, clove, cinnamon, lavender

St. John's All Purpose Salve: St. John's wort, calendula infused oils; essential oils of lavender and tea tree

Minor Scrapes (not to be used on deep cuts, gashes, or punctures): comfrey, yarrow, and calendula infused oils; essential oil of lavender

Cough Foot and Chest Rub: jojoba oil, mullein infused oil; essential oils of lavender, eucalyptus, cinnamon, rosemary, peppermint, ginger, thyme

Lip Balms - They Aren't Simply for Kids

Lip balms are the same basic recipe as salves with a few minor differences. You will still need 1 ounce of beeswax per 1 cup of carrier oil (even if you add cocoa butter, coconut oil, or shea butter). And you will only use 1-2 drops of essential oil per ¼ ounce container. Either small ¼ ounce salve containers or ¼ ounce tube lip balm containers work well here.

Warning: What not to use in lip balm:

- Arnica. Unless you have fat lip, arnica is not necessary on lips. Plus, it is usually a plant used for acute situations. As an oil, it stimulates circulation and is specific for inflammation, muscle and joint pain. So unless you get popped in the mouth, don't put arnica in lip balms.
- Essential oils to avoid in lip balms are spices, mints, and citrus oils. They are irritating to the lips. Some people think these are fine on lips and the irritating effects are counterbalanced by calendula or comfrey infused oil. That is sometimes true, but I recommend things that are more nourishing for constant use.

Carrier oils that are best for lip balms: jojoba oil, almond oil, grape seed oil, and avocado oil

Solid oils for lip balms: shea butter, coconut oil, and cocoa butter

Infused oils that are great for lip balms: calendula, comfrey root or leaf, plantain leaf

Some of my favorite essential oils for lip balms are lavender, chamomile, geranium or rosewood, vetiver or carrot seed essential oils. They are healing, soothing, and relaxing.

Chapter 5

A Series on Salts

Bath products made with salts are a vintage bath staple. They are, at times, seemingly simple, but they have never been a mere fad or waned in popularity.

Salts are magically packed with minerals from the earth or sea, the contents of which depend on where they hail from or what type of salt they are. The natural elements that combine to make salts have a healing power that is as important as any other element found in nature, making them an essential tool for health in any home or practice.

Salts are easy to work with and forgiving as a medium. They don't irritate the skin, and spilling them doesn't result in a big oily mess. You may use salts alone, but they also combine beautifully with essential oils and carrier oils to turn a basic bathtub into an instant home spa.

Scented salts can be aesthetically pleasing, infusing the air with scent and enriching the water with nutrients. They can also have potent medicinal effects. A salt with essential oil soak can soften skin, lessen inflammation in swollen muscles and joints, stimulate immunity, stop a spastic cough, induce sleep, or relax the heart and nervous system to a more harmonious place. One might even say, if willing to go there, that salts and healing baths also clear the energy field to facilitate soul and spiritual healing. But that is a topic for another book.

This chapter will outline how to produce different salt products for bath and body as well as what makes the salts used in these recipes such effective healing agents. Products you will learn to make are: bath salts, effervescent bath balls, salt scrubs, and smelling salts.

Each recipe will include the following: materials list, instructions for making, storage tips, shelf life and labeling. Sample plant formulas will be given at the end of the chapter, as they apply to all products included here.

Now, before we get to the making of products, let's explore what these small to microscopic crystals do, and how they do it!

Salts as Healers - How Do They Work?

Internally, salt (sodium chloride) is a mineral our bodies need to function daily and helps facilitate the absorption of nutrients. It is best consumed in unprocessed forms, such as sea salt, seaweed, celery, or other foods and herbs that have a significant amount of sodium balanced with other essential minerals.

Medicinally, salt, along with plants and food that contain salt, increase our cells' water content, which cools, relaxes, and calms metabolic and cellular function quickly. Salty things soften hard and dry tissues, help to clear lumps in the lymphatic system, and loosen phlegm that is dry and thick. The combination of salt's ability to moisten dry tissue and relax muscles is part of how they relieve constipation as well as tension in the respiratory tract.

As mentioned, salt softens irritation and dryness. In energetic herbal terms, we would say demulcent and emollient. These two words mean the same thing, but refer to different places in the body. Demulcent is to soften dry tissue internally, while emollient is to soften dry tissue externally.

Salt consumed in excess, though, has detrimental effects on health, causing one to retain fluids and build mass, thereby increasing heat and inflammation instead of cooling. High blood pressure and water retention are a few of the complications that arise with adverse effects on kidney, liver, and adrenal function.

When used for specific reasons, and by sticking with herbs and foods that are properly balanced in a natural way (i.e. by nature and not adulterated by processing), one can avoid these nasty side effects and reap the health benefits of the essential nutrient salt.

Epsom Salts

Epsom salts are magnesium salts. Magnesium is an essential mineral as well as an electrolyte. Internally, it supports proper nerve function, assists the movement of potassium and sodium in and out of cells, and works in tandem with calcium to maintain muscle function body wide. Calcium is responsible for muscle contraction, while magnesium triggers the muscle to relax. That goes for all muscles.

Magnesium as a supplement may reduce spasms of the heart and coronary arteries, reduce cholesterol, and inhibit platelet aggregation. I have also used it to relax simple muscle spasms in the neck, arms, legs, colon, and uterus. But I have also found that it successfully stops heart arrhythmias when tension from magnesium deficiency is exacerbating the symptom.

Externally, Epsom salts have similar uses. They are anti-inflammatory and work to warm and relax muscle and tissue to disperse heat and inflammation. They can be effective soaks for sprained body parts, general muscle soreness, and be helpful for some muscle pain and tension as a result of arthritis. They act as an anti-spasmodic and are specifically indicated for muscle spasms externally, not just internally. Epsom salts are also a potent drawing agent and are capable of drawing unwanted things from an area, be it pus and infection or clogged pores.

Note: Baths are contraindicated for high blood pressure. If you suffer from high blood pressure, please check with your doctor or a trained health professional before taking them for therapy.

In the recipe section for *Simple Bath Salts*, I will give more information on what to combine these salts with and suggestions for use.

Dead Sea Salts

The Dead Sea is a fresh water lake off the coast of Israel and Jordan. It rests over 1,200 feet below sea level. It is the lowest body of water on Earth, and has nearly four times the amount of salt as the ocean. The salt content is so high that it cannot support life, thus revealing its namesake. It can, however, support weight! Due to its high salt content, the Dead Sea is so buoyant that it can float a person and even prevent them from diving into or going under the water.

People have journeyed to the Dead Sea's coast for thousands of years to benefit from the healing and restorative powers the water, air, and mud possess. Historically, and to this day, salt and mud from the Dead Sea is specifically indicated for eczema, psoriasis, dermatitis, and arthritis. It may also help maintain a youthful appearance.

What makes the salt and mud from this specific location any different from other seas? Dead Sea salts contain nearly ten times the amount of minerals that ocean and other sea salts have. While ocean and sea salt contains around 80% sodium and sodium chloride, and 20% of other minerals, Dead Sea salt has about 35% sodium, with over 30 other supporting minerals, including magnesium, calcium, potassium, bromine, sulfur, and iodine. Each of these minerals has its individual benefits. As a whole, they assist cell metabolism, the absorption of nutrients, and the expulsion and elimination of waste products and toxins. They also act to lessen inflammation in tissue and muscle, and they support the health of hair, skin, and nails.

While Dead Sea salt is amazing, it is also more expensive. To offset the cost and reap the benefits, I often recommend that people mix Dead Sea salt with other salt. The therapy is still effective, but money and resources are saved.

Sea Salts

Sea salt doesn't compare to Dead Sea salt, but it is still an excellent second. It's great for the skin, having many of the same benefits and contents of Dead Sea salt, simply to less of a degree.

I find my favorite way to use sea salt, whether it's from the Himalayas or France, is combined with Epsom salts with a bit of Dead Sea salt thrown in.

Bath Salts

Manufacturing bath salts at home, like any product, is beneficial for plenty of reasons. Simple and inexpensive ingredients allow one to prepare them for a fraction of what you will pay for them retail while also having the benefit of tailoring them to a specific need or person. And assembling them is relatively easy with a short prep time, making them a great rainy day or birthday party craft project, gift, or something to whip up for a sudden acute illness.

Of course, you need to be prepared for that happy side effect of needing to take more baths. Taking more baths and making bath products isn't only for your health. Healing baths taken with home-prepared products can be an excellent teaching tool! In class, I teach how to make them, but I also encourage students to figure out different herbal formulas with salt combinations for specific needs.

Then I require them to take healing baths with their own salt formulas. Imagine, you're making bath salts, taking baths and enjoying yourself, but also learning loads about formulation, health, and the effects of herbal medicines.

Bath salt recipes can be basic, and may include only one essential oil with one basic salt. But I sometimes take pleasure in spicing them up by adding red clay and/or jojoba oil. The clay helps draw toxins from the skin, and the oil softens the skin while boosting essential oil absorption. It is not necessary to do this, though, in order to receive the benefits of the salts in the water, for the salts themselves make an excellent carrier.

Materials List

The list of things you need for bath salts is obvious. This list will include a few extras for more diverse formulation. Those items will be marked as optional. Your bath salt making station should/could include:

- Salts of choice: Dead Sea, Epsom, and/or sea salt
- Essential oils of choice
- Glass containers for storing. I prefer glass mason jars, because you can add your ingredients to the jar, shake to mix the salts, and store them as well.
- Stainless steel bowl for mixing *
- Stainless steel spoon for mixing *
- Glass or stainless steel measuring cup *
- Tablespoon
- Labels. I like Avery Labels from any place they sell office supplies. Or you can design your own!
- Carrier oils of choice, French clay (optional)

  *only needed if not using a mason jar

Instructions for Making and For Use

1. Add your salt/s of choice to the mason jar or the mixing bowl. This may be a combination of equal parts Dead Sea salt, sea salt, and Epsom salt, or simply one. It's your choice.

2. Per 1 cup of salts, add 35-40 drops of essential oils. **Warning**: *Don't use citrus or spices! They will irritate the skin, causing rashes.*
3. Optional: mix in 2 tablespoons of clay and 2 tablespoons of carrier oil per single cup of salt.
4. Put the lid on and shake the jar to combine the ingredients.
5. Store away from heat and out of the sun, as this will cause rancidity. For optimal scent absorption, let sit for a few weeks before using or giving as a gift.

To use: Add approximately ¼- ½ cup of the salts to your bath, soak and enjoy! Then repeat! Multiple uses are what deem the process medicinal.

Storage Tips, Shelf Life, and Labeling

Storage: Storing bath salts is fairly simple. As stated in the instructions, keep them in an airtight container, away from heat, and out of direct sunlight. You may wish to use a colored glass container, but it's not necessary if you have a lightless place to keep them.

Shelf life: These stay shelf stable for about 8-12 weeks. If you use carrier oil in them (i.e. almond, grape seed, etc.), they will go rancid in 4-6 weeks. Jojoba oil will not cause rancidity, but it does make the salts sticky and messy after about 4-6 weeks. I therefore assign a shelf life of 4-6 weeks for jojoba oil salts, too. The hope is that you take many baths and use these salts up quickly.

Labeling: Label everything! Write the following: date made, shelf life, all of the product's ingredients, product name and uses (if you're getting creative), instructions for use (especially if this is a gift), and the shelf life.

I highly recommend you keep notes on what you made, how you did it (especially if you deviate from special instructions), and what you put into it. Why? This will help you determine what you may want to repeat or change.

Lavender Lemongrass Epsom Salt Bath

I'm a big fan of healing baths. And salt baths are one of my favorites. Salts are known for their restorative powers. While it's nice to get fancy and use different combinations of sea salt, Dead Sea salt, or pink salt, that can get expensive. I've found that simple Epsom salts make an excellent carrier for essential oils in the tub. They are easy to find and relatively inexpensive.

This bath formula is one of my favorites, and includes essential oils of lavender and lemongrass in an Epsom salt and almond oil base. It is harmonizing to the heart, nervous system, and immune system. It has the ability to bring balance, allowing one to root into a healing process or just calm down in the wake of a stressful period. I have found it to also be an excellent bath formula for those recovering from illness or suffering from muscle aches associated with the flu, bronchitis, or other respiratory infections that cause muscle strain from coughing too much.

Ingredients and Preparation

- 4 cups of Epsom salts or salt of choice
- 1 tablespoon of lavender pure essential oil
- 1 tablespoon of lemongrass pure essential oil
- 2 ounces of almond oil

Making this is very simple. Take all the ingredients, put them in the bowel or jar, and mix or shake. Dispense into your containers for gifting or storing, and label. With salts, it is best to let them sit in a cool dark place for 3-5 days before using. The essential oils will better infuse the salts. In this case it is not necessary, for the almond oil will help this process.

To make herbal gifts, you don't have to be a professional herbalist. You just have to know your limits. Choose good simple recipes with clear instructions. Be sure to read up on the plants you plan to use, and be sure those plants have few to no contraindications.

Effortless Effervescent Bath Balls

Years ago I got a gift from one of my music students. It was a package of balls called "Bath Bombs," a name I found offensive. Who wanted to bomb their bath? Regardless, I wanted to know what these were. That night, I filled the tub to try one out. As I removed a purple ball from the package, the stench of synthetic fragrance wafted my way. Unappealing as this was, curiosity won, and in the tub it went.

The ball hit the water and immediately exploded into a fizzing mass. I was intrigued. As I watched it dissolve into effervescent nothingness, I thought, "I can make that."

After making note of a few active ingredients, I began to play. There were plenty of failed attempts, but eventually I had bath balls. Unlike the others, these were all natural, free of additives, preservatives, food coloring, and synthetic fragrances.

And because these are easy to make, as well as fun to use, they are an excellent kids craft for a rainy day.

Materials List and Recipe

- Measuring spoons and glass measuring cups
- Receptacle for heating the solid fat
- Glass container for storing product
- 1 cup of baking soda
- ½ cup of citric acid
- 2 tablespoons of cornstarch
- 5 tablespoons of coconut oil (or shea butter)
- 2 tablespoons of carrier oil of choice (almond, jojoba, apricot seed, etc.)
- 40 drops total of essential oil (1 to 2 oils)

Instructions For Making and For Use

1. Warm the coconut oil on low. I usually use my glass Pyrex or stainless steel measuring cup for this. I simply add the fat to the cup, set the cup in a saucepan with water, and turn it on low.

2. While it is melting, put the baking soda, citric acid, and cornstarch together in a stainless steel bowl. Mix them together well.

3. Once the coconut oil is liquefied, add your carrier oil of choice to it. Let them sit together while the two reach the same temperature. This will prevent the coconut oil from hardening too quickly when you add the fat to the dry contents.

4. Add the liquefied fat to the dry ingredients. Mix.

5. Add the essential oils and mix well. At this point, if more liquid is needed mix in some carrier oil in 1/2 teaspoon increments (and don't add more then 1 ½ teaspoons total). The goal is that balls should pack together and hold their shape without falling apart.

6. Now make the balls. Take a tablespoon of the mix and work it in your hand until you have formed a ball. Set them on a plate or stainless steel tray to dry and harden. This recipe makes approximately 25 balls.

Instructions for use: add 2-3 balls per bath and stay in the tub for at least 20 minutes.

Storage Tips, Shelf Life, and Labeling

Storage: Store these in a glass jar with a lid, out of sunlight and away from heat.

Shelf Life: If you used jojoba oil, these can keep well for 2-3 months. If you didn't, however, their shelf life is 4-6 weeks.

Labeling: Yes, this is a repeat. Because I have found people need to read things many times. Label everything! Write the following: date made and, shelf life, all of the products ingredients, product name and uses (if you're getting creative), instructions for use (especially if this is a gift), and the shelf life.

I highly recommend you keep notes on what you made, how you did it (especially if you deviate from special instructions), and what you put into it. Why? This will help you determine what you may want to repeat or change in the future.

A Re-tooled Classic: Smelling Salts

According to chemist, Bob Trach, "Smelling salts are made of ammonium carbonate, a colorless to white crystalline powder. Ammonium carbonate is mixed with a perfume to create a stimulant. The ammonia fumes from the salts trigger membranes of the nose and lungs, which initiate a reflex to cause the muscles that control breathing to work faster."

Smelling salts have been traced back thousands of years, as far as Ancient Roman times. While they are specifically ammonium carbonate and used to stimulate respiration, the salts we will be making will be used for different reasons and with less caustic and dangerous materials.

I began making smelling salts for headaches, coughs, mental stimulation, nausea, and relaxation. They are a quick and easy way to incorporate medicinal aromatherapy into your day. Smelling salts can be carried in small containers and used liberally without offending others in a small office space, work environment, or airplane. And if they spill, there is a small mess of salt, not a big mess of oil – big plus!

Materials List

- Essential oils of choice
- Chunky sea salt
- Small bottle or vial (¼ ounce in size)

Instructions for Making and For Use

Fill the bottle ¾ of the way full with sea salt. Add 6 drops total of essential oil.

Now use it! I often recommend people take a five minute break from their work, step outside or just outside of their work space, and inhale their smelling salts for five minutes. If on a plane, and you're using the salts for panic disorder, use liberally.

Storage Tips, Shelf Life, and Labeling

Storage Tips: None special.

Shelf Life: As long as you need them.

Labeling: Still, as stated in the above recipes. Label everything!

Body Scrubs

This luxury item is easy to produce, but it takes a bit more effort to use, and a lot of salt. Therefore, it's not as inexpensive as others, but it is worth it. When you use the scrub, you're emulating a spa experience.

The health benefits are greater than other bath products. You stimulate the tactile sense of touch, which is good for the skin and the nerves. This blend of salts and oils also aids the leaching of toxins from the skin, balances the tone of the skin, and makes the skin soft. If you like, purchase an all-natural loofah sponge to intensify the scrub even more.

Materials List

These materials will be enough to make a pint of scrub. You are welcome to double or triple the recipe.

- Coffee grinder
- Large glass container
- Stainless steel spoon for mixing
- 2 ¼ cups total of Epsom salts, Dead Sea salts, and/or sea salts (the combination and amount of each is up to you)
- 1 teaspoon total of essential oils of your choice
- ¾ cup of carrier oil (jojoba, almond, apricot, grape seed, etc.)

Instructions for Making and For Use

1. Grind the salts in the coffee grinder. You may use a normal sized kitchen grinder. When I was making them in quantities to sell, I purchased a large one for $50 at Bed Bath & Beyond.
2. Add the salts to the jar.
3. Add the carrier oil and essential oils.
4. Stir gently and then put a lid on it for storage.

Stand in the bathtub or on a bath towel, and before stepping into the shower or settling into the tub, scoop out and scrub legs and body with the mixture. Apply wherever you can reach.

Note: Avoid scrubbing varicose veins, bruises, or irritated skin.

Warning: *Please beware that oil makes the tub slippery. Be safe.*

Storage Tips, Shelf Life, and Labeling

Storage Tips: Please see recipe for Effervescent Bath Balls.

Shelf Life: 4-6 weeks away from sunlight and heat.

Labeling: Please see recipe for Effervescent Bath Balls.

Sample Plant Formulas for Products Listed

Warming and Stimulating (not relaxing to most): rosemary and clove

Balancing and Anxiety Relieving: lemongrass and lavender

Immune Support & Emotional Harmonizer: lavender, lemongrass, and vetiver

Feet on the Ground: frankincense and vetiver

Intoxicating Rose: rosewood, cardamom, and clary sage

PMS relief: clary sage and lavender

Respiratory Health: frankincense and clove

Anti-fungal: geranium and clove

Immune Herbal Immersion: lavender and thyme

Muscle Madness (includes overuse, flu, or rib pain from excessive coughing): Epsom salts, lavender, lemongrass, clove, or rosemary (small amount)

Chapter 6

Healing Hands Cream

Creature comforts are important, and one of my favorites is a silky pot of body cream. It soothes skin, envelops the senses, and makes one feel rich and pampered. The problem is that products purchased in the store are dissatisfying, with even the "natural" products tending to be lackluster. They also often contain ingredients that don't agree with sensitive skin and are extremely expensive.

My rekindled affinity for skin care products was brought on by an awareness of my own skin. Age, stress, autoimmune disease, weather, and life circumstances have been hard on it. Frankly, I'm also rather lazy about caring for it, which doesn't help. But there is a hook that keeps me mostly engaged. And that is – when my skin feels good, so do I.

My own awareness has inspired me to retool an old skin cream recipe that I used to market. I have fashioned it to be flexible, allowing the maker to choose different herb teas, essential and infused oils specific to their skins needs. It is fairly simple to make, and it whips up silky smooth with a scent that is divine. It is medicinal yet decadent. I call it *Healing Hands Cream*, for it puts the power to heal in your hands. Despite its name, it may be used on any body part.

The Skin's Role as an Organ

The skin is our largest organ, and we wear it on the outside. It takes 14-18 square feet of it to cover our adult bodies and holds down a job as measurably large, if not larger. It is an organ that is the first physical part of us to meet our world, and is in charge of body regulation from the inside out. Some of its important duties:

- It is an organ of elimination, keeping in balance how our body deals with waste.
- It is a sensory organ, informing our internal workings of changes in our environment and pain.
- It synthesizes vitamin D, excretes oil, salt and water via sweat to regulate temperature and help detoxify our body.

> It is a voice for internal organ and endocrine system dysfunction by displaying rashes, acne, pigment discoloration, eczema, etc.
> As if those responsibilities were not enough, the skin is part of our immune system, protecting our internal world from many hazards by baring infection, ultraviolet rays, and toxins.

The condition of our skin and its health is affected greatly by our life experiences and choices, such as how and where we live, what we eat, hormones, age, and disease. It takes working from the inside out to fully support the skin when deficiency arises. But working from the outside in is just as important. You see, medicinal agents can absorb through the skin and into the bloodstream, traveling to internal destinations to heal and help maintain balance while also relieving topical irritation.

Book Recommendation: The importance of medicines applied through the skin is further highlighted by the work of French herbalist, Maurice Mésségué. In his practice, he prescribes herbal hand and foot baths to his clients for their ailments. His philosophy is well illustrated in his informative and entertaining book, *Of Plants and People*.

Basic Cream Recipe

If you've read the chapter on salves and infusions and tried your hand at them, you will quickly see that creams are a bit more involved. But with the few simple tricks I will give you here, yours should turn out beautifully. The recipe is written to make about 11 ounces of cream.

What follows is: An ingredients and tools list, instructions for making the basic cream, and options for plants used based on symptom pictures.

Ingredients list

- 2 ounces solid fat (or shea butter)
- 3 ounces infused oil (calendula or comfrey), or almond oil
- 2 ounces jojoba - as a natural preservative
- 2-3 ounces purified water, rose water, or an herbal tea

- 1/8 teaspoon of boric acid (optional, see notes)
- 1/2 teaspoon of plain goat yogurt (optional, see notes)
- 1 ounce beeswax
- 10 drops essential oil if desired

Facts on Ingredients:

> Jojoba oil acts as a natural preservative and is actually a wax distilled from a bean. It has an oily consistency. Add 15-20% jojoba oil to a recipe for this effect. This method will not work as well if your product has a higher content of water, and is a lotion instead of a cream. Lotions are okay, but a natural lotion will mold quickly. Just be aware of that.

> Boric acid can be found as Borax in the laundry section at the your local hardware store, co-op, grocer, or Target. It is a salt compound found in dry salt lakebeds, in food and soil. It contains boron, oxygen, and hydrogen. It is anti-septic and makes your cream whiter. You may choose not to use it if you like, but it is quite safe to use.

> Plain goat yogurt added to the cream facilitates the emulsification of fat and water. Because oil and water want to separate, adding an emulsifier makes them mix to create a single consistency. Other natural emulsifiers that you may find in your fridge are egg and mayonnaise. Goat yogurt, though, is my favorite.

If you need to avoid dairy, one could also use soya lecithin. I don't use soya lecithin because many people are allergic to soy.

Of course, there are some that cannot use either. If this is the case, simply rely on agitation for emulsification, and beeswax to help aid the setting of your creams consistency. If you have a high content of water in your cream, making it more a lotion, there will be separation when the product sits. To remix, simply shake before each use.

Products that have water in them and separate often will mold more easily. I find using an emulsifier creates a product that is more shelf stable.

Tools

Other supplies you will need are:

- Kitchen scale
- Double boiler
- Stainless steel tablespoon
- Small glass containers to pour/spoon the cream into once complete
- Hand mixer or blender (may also mix in a large stainless steel bowl)
- Labels

My own personal tip: I use a stainless steel measuring cup in a saucepan with water for a double boiler when preparing small batches. To mix, I use a hand held mixer inserted into the cup instead of a blender. I find it easier to clean.

Jars and containers for creams come in glass or plastic and in an array of sizes. I like to make them in 2 or 4 ounce sizes, and smaller ones for portable creams.

Instructions for Making

1. Measure your liquid oil, and add it to the double boiler. Then, weigh your shea butter and beeswax on the scale, and add it to the oil.

2. Melt the shea butter and beeswax into the oil on low heat. Use a stainless steel spoon to stir until blended. Remove from heat.

3. Warm the water or herb tea with the boric acid or soya lecithin (do not boil). If using boric acid, be sure it totally dissolves.

Important tip: Warming the water helps it emulsify better with the hot fat and wax mixture you have.

4. Put water into a mixing bowl or blender and agitate with an electric mixer or turn blender on. If you didn't use soya lecithin, now is the time to add the goat yogurt. As the water spins, slowly pour the oil mixture in. Mix until emulsified.

5. Add in the essential oils at the end. Mix slightly and then put cream into containers. Allow it to cool before attaching the lid.

Storage Tips, Shelf Life and Labeling

Storage Tips: Just as before, store out of sunlight and away from heat in glass or plastic jars. I use glass for home and plastic for travel. Also, avoid humid environments.

Shelf Life: If you used 20% jojoba oil and 2 ounces of water, as given in these instructions, your cream will store up to a year without a problem, as long as you keep it away from sunlight and heat. The more water you use, the shorter shelf life your product will have.

Signs that there is something amiss with your product: Does it smell bad? Has the color changed? Is there mold growing on it? Does it feel and look unusual?

Labeling: Date each jar and make note of any changes you made to the recipe and the plants you used.

Sample Formulas for Creams

As promised, here are my recommendations based on symptom pictures for skin. I'm avoiding anything too detoxifying or pushy here. This cream is to nurture.

Remember, if you are making a tea or marshmallow root infusion, make it strong enough to have effect. For herb tea, use 1 tablespoon steeped in 3 ounces hot water for 10 minutes. To make the marshmallow root decoction, it takes a bit longer. Place 1 tablespoon of the root in 3 ounces of water and let it sit overnight. Be sure when you press out your tea/decoction you still have 3 ounces. Add a little more water post press if needed.

Tight dry skin: Tea of marshmallow root, plantain leaf; Infused oil of calendula or comfrey; Essential oils of vetiver, frankincense.

Burning and itching skin: Tea of marshmallow root or plantain leaf; Infused oil of calendula flower and plantain leaf, St. John's wort; Essential oils of lavender, vetiver.

Dry and red skin: Tea of chamomile, or marshmallow root decoction; Infused oil of comfrey leaf and plantain leaf; Essential oils of vetiver, geranium, or rose.

Aging skin: Tea of rose water; Infused oil of calendula flower and comfrey leaf; Essential oils of rose, frankincense, vetiver.

Oily skin: Tea of rosemary; Essential oils of lemongrass, juniper, and lavender for balance.

Damp skin w/ lack of tonicity: Tea of sage; Essential oils of rose geranium, sage, lavender.

Making your own skin cream has many benefits. For one, you know what you are putting on and in your body. Secondly, you have a skin care plan that is tailored to your specific needs, making for a more effective use of time and resources. And thirdly, you save money! It costs tons less to make 11 ounces of cream than to purchase something natural that you would want to use. And it makes an amazing gift.

Chapter 7

Simple Essential Oil Sprays for Hands, Health, and Home

Could it get any easier than putting a few things in a bottle, labeling, shaking, and spraying? Not really. And the benefits are profound. I use sprays at home to sanitize the carpets and furniture (especially after illness), clear the air (think bathroom), use as hand sanitizer (in lieu of chemicals), and sometimes for cleaning.

Materials

What you need is simple.

- Glass bottles with spray pumps. The bottles with spray pumps come in glass, amber brown or cobalt blue, and can be found in 1, 2, or 4 ounce sizes.
- Essential oils of your choice
- Witch hazel
- Distilled water
- Labels

Instructions

1. First, add 1 part witch hazel to 1 part distilled water. If you are making a 4 ounce size, that is 2 ounces of witch hazel and 2 ounces of water.
2. Add 3-6 drops total of essential oil per ounce of this base. In a 4 ounce bottle, that is 12-24 drops total.
3. Put the lid on. Shake before each use.

Label with a date and the ingredients used. This will keep indefinitely.

Sample Formulas

Mystic Medley: frankincense, myrrh, sweet mandarin, clove

Holiday Spice: clove, cinnamon, cardamom, sweet mandarin

Anti-infectious: lavender, thyme, cinnamon, vetiver

Kid Friendly Suggestion: For fear of monsters, I came up with this one about 20 years ago. It's called *Monster-Be-Gone Bedtime Spray* and includes lavender, sweet mandarin, and lemongrass. It eradicates monsters. To make it, follow the instructions above, but cut the amount of essential oils in half.

Section 2

Applications: Chapters 8-10

Chapter 8

Herbs for Acute Respiratory Infections

Acute Illness and the Respiratory Tract

The respiratory tract is the most highly infected area in the body, with many healthy adults and children experiencing 4-8 acute infections per year. The duration and severity of these infections vary according to the person and the illness. For example, the common cold may last 5-10 days, while bronchitis can drag on for three weeks or more.

An acute illness differs from a chronic illness in that it comes on suddenly, runs its course fairly quickly, and resolves. They can result from a viral, bacterial, or fungal infection. In this chapter, I'll be addressing viral and bacterial infections.

Some common acute infections of the upper respiratory tract are sinusitis, colds, influenza, laryngitis, croup, tonsillitis, strep throat, and whooping cough. A few of the lower respiratory tract infections are bronchitis, pneumonia, and RSV (Respiratory Syncytial Virus – a viral infection of the lungs and respiratory passage that affects toddlers).

Acute illness comes with the territory of being human. But many people would love to eradicate these viral and bacterial infections altogether, because each illness ensures that the sufferer is inconvenienced, uncomfortable, and sometimes bedridden.

While these pesky bugs are tiresome, they may also serve a purpose. When we're sick, we are forced to rest and listen to our body differently, taking a beneficial break. I also believe that illness makes us stronger. Each passing year we are challenged to survive new strains of virus and bacteria, stress and disease. Our body and immune system must become heartier and smarter in order to navigate these strange and constantly mutating waters. The learning process that is facilitated by the virus or bacteria combined with healthy food choices (eating the healthiest we can afford to), getting decent sleep, and taking time off to enjoy life can strengthen us, providing a good foundation for our future health.

When we are plagued with acute illness, or coming upon the season where they are most active, herbs support us in multiple ways. They can safely and effectively help us manage symptoms, support the immune response, act as nutritional tonics, and help create a terrain that doesn't support illness.

To help you learn how to use plant medicines effectively, I will map out how to formulate (put plants together) for different respiratory infections and their symptoms. I will also list and define energetics (actions of plants) associated with the illnesses, and list plants with those energetics.

Warning: Please know that the following information is not intended to diagnose conditions or to prescribe herbs. That is illegal. By law, doctors, nurse practitioners, and physician's assistants are the only ones who are allowed to diagnose and prescribe. I always recommend that if you are very ill, not responding to treatment, and/or in doubt, please consult a physician.

Formulation

A formula is a group of two or more plants that we use in combination to address a health issue. While there are times a simple (a single plant) is appropriate, the complex symptom picture presented by an acute illness typically needs a formula.

Formulating can be a detailed process, but I'll try to keep my advice simple and to the point.

> ➤ When suffering from an infection, we want some relief. Chose herbs that are specific to your symptom picture. For example, if there is a bone chilling high fever, be sure to include a relaxing diaphoretic (fever reducer) in your treatment plan, such as boneset, yarrow, or blue vervain. If there are profuse wet secretions with postnasal drip accompanied by a sore throat and low-grade fever, consider something astringent that dries excess moisture, but slightly moistens by bringing up oil, and is a mild diaphoretic, such as sage.

➤ Choose plants that support the organs of elimination to ensure the toxins released by bacterial or viral die off are appropriately excreted. This often happens naturally, as many of the plants we use are diuretic (increasing urination) and bitter (stimulating to the liver). Often, this requirement is fulfilled by the simple addition of more teas and water.

➤ Include a good lymphatic to support the body's fight. The lymphatic system houses the immune system. It includes plants such as echinacea, calendula, cleavers, and poke root, to name a few. Some of these are also anti-bacterial and immune potentiating. Refer to the list of energetics for more information on that.

➤ Don't forget anti-viral and/or anti-bacterial plants. They work to shorten the duration of the illness. They can also protect us from contracting a secondary bacterial or viral infection. People with immune systems compromised by disease, medications, smoking, stress, or those who often suffer from recurrent acute infections in winter do well to include these.

➤ Be sure to know when to use something to calm the nerves. Our body's immune system works best when we are relaxed, and, better yet, sleeping. Certain individuals may tend towards agitation, especially if you have a high fever or a spastic cough. So give the nervous and immune system a break with a good nervine. Most of the diaphoretics (fever reducers) are excellent nervines, but it's something to be conscious of. Essential oils may also be an indispensible tool here.

There are times when an illness will respond immediately to an herbal protocol and times when the response is slower, because herbs don't work as quickly as drugs. Map out a plan. If you experience gradual relief and are managing symptoms, you are probably on the right track.

If you feel the formula is ineffective, and there has been little symptom relief after 1-2 days, change a plant or two instead of chucking the whole. When making this change, observe and remember the four qualities. And remember, you can do the right thing, but there is still a chance that what you have chosen may not work predictably. In this instance, simply try again.

If after 3-4 days you feel yourself worsening or unable to turn a corner, call for help. You may have contracted a secondary illness. As stated before, consult with a doctor if you are concerned, especially if the fever is rising, you are at risk of dehydration, or you're having difficulty breathing.

Energetics and the Herbs that Support Them

In Chapter 1, I mentioned that energetic terms are those that describe a plant's action on the body. Below you will find the ones most commonly applied when treating acute respiratory infections. Each term is defined, and a list of plants that have the desired effect is given. Specific information on what plants to consider when formulating will be found under each symptom and illness.

Also remember that when making a formula for symptoms and the illness, it is essential to consider whether the plant is warming, cooling, drying, or moistening, and in some cases relaxing or stimulating. I will provide some guidance on that throughout this chapter as well as in the *Materia medica*.

Anti-bacterial: These are herbs that take direct action against bacteria. They are not nearly as strong as antibiotics. Examples are usnea, calendula, sage, thyme, goldenseal, garlic, oregano, and cinnamon.

Anti-fungal: These substances act to kill off fungus. Examples are barberry, cardamom, thyme, usnea, calendula, Oregon grape root, and myrrh.

Anti-histamine: Histamines are released due to an allergic reaction, making cell walls inflamed, permeable, easily irritated, and profusely runny/leaky; anti-histamines inhibit their release and relieve inflammation and irritation. Examples are peppermint, elderberry, and nettle leaf tincture.

Anti-inflammatory: These reduce inflammation and irritation. In this case, they can be useful for headaches that accompany fevers or to reduce the inflammation produced by the heat. Their action is contingent on their ability to reduce symptoms without disabling the immune system. Excellent anti-inflammatory herbs for fevers are ginger, peppermint, yarrow, blue vervain, lavender, linden blossom, sage, and chamomile.

Anti-infective: These herbs improve the body's own defenses against germs or parasites. They may be used when one is exposed to a pathogen to prevent infection or to shorten the duration or severity of the illness. Excellent anti-infective agents are echinacea, ginger, yarrow, lavender, sage, and hyssop.

Anti-microbial or anti-septic: These are plants that inhibit the proliferation of a virus or bacteria and stimulate the body's innate ability to recover. Excellent plants in this scope are cinnamon, echinacea, elderberry, ginger, goldenseal, holy basil, thyme, usnea, and yarrow.

Anti-spasmodics, muscular: These relieve spasms in muscles and the tension and constriction that result from spasms, as applied to acute illness, intestinal, stomach or coughing spasms. Examples are chamomile, ginger, wild cherry bark, marshmallow root (mild), plantain, skullcap (when nerve related), black cohosh, passionflower, motherwort, hawthorn, black haw and cramp bark, lobelia, mullein leaf, catnip, and peppermint.

Anti-spasmodics, nerve: These relieve spasms and ticks that occur as a result of constriction and irritation of the nerves. Examples are California poppy, passionflower, skullcap, peppermint, and lemon balm.

Anti-viral: These take direct action against viruses. Please note that plants generally have an affinity for certain viruses. Refer to your *Materia medica* for those specifics. Examples are cinnamon, licorice root, lemon balm, thyme, yarrow, basil, and oregano.

Astringents: These tighten mucous membranes, thereby decreasing inflammation in the tissue. This provides a barrier, preventing leakage out or large molecules getting in. Useful for diarrhea, hemorrhoids, and runny noses, to name a few. Examples are echinacea, raspberry leaf, sage, and yarrow.

Bronchodilators: These are agents that dilate or open the bronchi and airway to increase air passage to the lungs; they are extremely useful in cases of RSV and bronchitis, or any time an airway passage has become constricted. Examples are Chinese ephedra (a.k.a. ma huang, which is now illegal and not available to the general public), strong black coffee (may add raw honey), and American ephedra.

Carminatives: These are herbs that relieve spasms and gas in the intestinal tract and gut; they are often anti-spasmodics in the respiratory tract, and some are diaphoretics. Examples are chamomile, peppermint, yarrow, cardamom, holy basil, fenugreek, ginger, and thyme.

Circulatory stimulants: These warm the body by warming and stimulating the blood and immune response. This is necessary when acute illness becomes a chronic problem in winter. Examples are cardamom, cinnamon, garlic, ginger, and elderberry.

Decongestants: These relieve mucus congestion in the sinuses and upper respiratory tract. Examples are peppermint, rosemary, thyme, horseradish, cayenne, ginger.

Demulcents: These sooth irritated mucus membranes, and, though most practitioners don't profess, are also anti-inflammatory. They should be used in cases of dry and wet spastic coughs (see under "Coughs" in the next section for details). Examples are slippery elm, marshmallow root, licorice root, plantain, mullein leaf, garlic, and fenugreek.

Diaphoretics: These are plants that increase the temperature of the body and stimulate the circulatory system to bring on a sweat and relieve a fever. They may also relax tension in the nervous system to increase circulation to the periphery and open the skin's pores to bring on a sweat and relieve a fever. Relaxant acrid bitters are blue vervain, calendula, catnip, linden blossom, lavender, and yarrow. Stimulating aromatic pungent diaphoretics are *Angelica archangelica*, calendula, echinacea, holy basil, ginger, elderflower, and sage.

Expectorant: This is a substance that thins and dries and/or stimulates the release of mucus from the lungs and bronchial mucosa. Examples are licorice root, ginger, marshmallow root, plantain, red root, thyme, slippery elm bark, elecampane, yerba santa, and osha.

Immune modulators/stimulants: These work to stimulate white blood cell counts and other processes of the immune system that support us in warding off illness. Recommended immune stimulants are echinacea, ginger, and elderberry.

Lymphatics: These plants increase the circulation of lymphatic fluid, thereby relieving lymph inflammation (swollen glands included); they can also improve immune function and act as anti-inflammatories in other parts of the body, depending on which plant you use. Examples are echinacea, burdock root, red root, cleavers, calendula, and poke root.

Mucosal anti-inflammatory: These reduce inflammation and histamine production in mucus membranes. This reduces the amount of mucus in the sinus and respiratory tract. There are times when this problem alone is triggering a cough. Support can be found from hyssop, eyebright, peppermint, and sage.

Nervines for acute illness: These are relaxing to the nervous system; many are also diaphoretic and anti-microbial. Examples are chamomile, lavender, skullcap, lemon balm, blue vervain, yarrow, cleavers, and calendula.

Applicable Strategies and Plants for Acute Illnesses and Symptoms

Below is an alphabetical list of symptoms and infections. I will give strategies and sample formulas for dealing with each.

- Bronchitis
- Colds
- Conjunctivitis
- Coughs
- Croup
- Earaches
- Fevers
- Flu
- Headaches
- Sedatives
- Sinus Congestion and Inflammation
- Sinusitis
- Sore Throat

- Stomach Virus
- Swollen Lymph Nodes/Glands; Mononucleosis

Bronchitis

Bronchitis is a viral infection that causes inflammation in the mucosal lining in the bronchial tubes. As described by Mary Bove, N.D. in her wonderful book, *An Encyclopedia of Natural Healing for Infants and Children*, the beginning symptoms of bronchitis look much like a cold. You may have a runny nose, low-grade fever, and slight dry cough. After about three days, however, the middle phase begins, as the infection moves deeper into the lungs, manifesting as a spastic, harsh, irritated, dry, and painful cough with a fever that rises. Some in the middle phase also have irritation with wheezing and a profuse amount of mucous.

The bronchitis cough can be extremely persistent. Due to its intensity, there may be vomiting or pain in the rib cage due to a pulled muscle.

Once the infection subsides, the cough becomes less painful with easier expectoration, but can still linger for up to three weeks.

Energetics to support bronchitis are anti-inflammatory, anti-viral, anti-bacterial, expectorants (for wet cough, choose stimulating; for dry cough, choose relaxing), diaphoretics, and demulcent.

Beginning symptoms: runny nose, low-grade fever, and cough.

Treat as you would a cold. At this point, most people don't realize they have bronchitis unless they are sure they have been exposed, or they are prone to bronchitis.

Middle symptoms: dry hacking cough that does not cease, or a wet hacking cough that does not cease, moderately high fever, wheezing, bronchial irritation, and inflammation.

Dry cough tincture formula (in a 60 ml or 2 ounce bottle): 10 ml lobelia, 15 ml elecampane root and/or 15 ml licorice root (*Glycyerrhiza glabra*), 10 ml Solomon's seal root, 10 ml echinacea or calendula.

Dry cough teas: marshmallow root or plantain leaf, grindelia, thyme, honey. Add 1 ounce each of grindelia and thyme.

Wet irritated cough tincture formula: 10 ml lobelia, 20 ml elecampane, horehound.

Wet irritated cough tea formula: mullein leaf (make it in a tea bag so the hairs don't irritate the throat), ginger root with honey.

Wet and over productive cough (as a tea): elecampane, pleurisy root, thyme, ginger root, and lobelia. Use 1 ounce of each plant, and ¼ ounce of lobelia to 1½ quarts of water.

Unless you have a wet over-productive cough in the middle phase, avoid anything heating or drying.

Later symptoms: cough may loosen and expectorate easier; fever abates.

Same tincture as for dry cough, but add in ginger if expectoration becomes very wet.

Post infection tincture and tea formulas (a formula for a cough that persists):

10 ml lobelia, 15 ml licorice root or elecampane, 35 ml Solomon's seal root – 35 drops 3 times daily. For ages 3-6, cut the dosage in half.

Tea formula for the wet and over productive cough: elecampane, ginger root, and thyme. Use 1/4 ounce of each plant to 1½ quarts of water.

Tea formula for the dry and irritated cough: plantain leaf, thyme, and elecampane root. Use ¼ ounce of each plant to 1½ quarts of water.

Wheezing:

This symptom requires a bronchodilator. I have had great success at home and with clients using coffee. It is not only effective in adults but also with children who have RSV or other lower respiratory infections. Children ages 1-3 can take 1 teaspoon every 5-10 minutes until symptoms abate, or as needed. It works well to increase air passage to the lungs. I have seen these kids recuperate quicker and be better able to eat and drink as well. For kids over age four, use 2 teaspoons to 2 tablespoons as needed. For adults, be your own dosage judge, but don't overdo it. You want to rest and not be over stimulated by caffeine.

Colds

Colds are often thought of as literally being cold in the body that is aggravated by wind. Colds need heat, so use warm and stimulating diaphoretics to heat the body. A strong and steamy cup of ginger tea with honey can assist the fight of the common cold very well, for example. It helps dry wetness, warms the blood, is anti-inflammatory, and acts as a potent diaphoretic.

Classic cold symptoms: low fever, aversion to cold sometimes with the inability to sweat, clear runny nose, white coating on tongue, itchy sore throat, congestion, coughing, post nasal drip, malaise, sneezing, and headache. It is also not unusual to experience swollen lymph glands, earaches, and watery eyes.

When formulating, please remember to take into account dry, wet, hot, and cold. What are you experiencing? Review the *Formulation* section above. When formulating for colds, unless it has become a recurring infection (one that doesn't resolve after having it once, but continues to return), I keep formulas simple, using just 2-3 plants and a tea or two.

Colds can become bronchitis, pneumonia, croup, sinusitis, or laryngitis. If your fever begins to rise above low-grade, you may be coming down with one of these.

Tinctures for Colds:

Sinus support: elecampane, horseradish, and thyme

Lung support: elecampane, licorice, thyme, plantain, osha, ginger

Lymphatic: echinacea, calendula

Too much wetness: sage, eyebright, ginger, peppermint, and yarrow

Irritation: sage, echinacea, plantain

Moistening: plantain, marshmallow root, and mullein leaf

Low-grade fever: yarrow, catnip

Note: Many of the tinctures above are diaphoretics.

Low-grade fever teas: ginger tea, yarrow and catnip tea, sage leaf tea, and elderflower tea

Wetness and irritation: sage leaf and yarrow tea

Aromatherapy Formula:

Eucalyptus globulus, thyme, lavender

This formula can be made in a carrier oil and applied to the neck, chest, and feet. You might also like to use a drop or two of these oils in a steam. See the *Sinus* section for instructions.

Conjunctivitis

Conjunctivitis, also known as pink eye, is an inflammation of the mucous membrane on the eye surface (called the conjunctiva). The pink begins in the corner of the eye near the nose and spreads from there. The infection can be bacterial or viral. In the bacterial infection, a dark yellow-green goo will be excreted from the eye, and the fever will be high. Viral responds to herbs quickly, and the mucous that comes from the eye is yellowish.

Eye Drops:

Basic tea for eye drops: eyebright and fennel. In 8 ounces of water, add 2 teaspoons of each. Let steep for 10 minutes and cool before use. Use a dropper to apply 4-6 times daily.

For bacterial conjunctivitis, add 10 drops of goldenseal glycerin tincture to the tea.

For viral conjunctivitis, add 10 drops of echinacea tincture.

Tincture for Internal Use:

Tincture formula: equal parts of calendula, cleavers, echinacea, and goldenseal or usnea. Take about 5-15 drops of this formula 3-4 times daily.

Herb Tea for Internal Use:

Yarrow and calendula (add eyebright if very wet, and honey if you like).

Note: Bacterial conjunctivitis may need antibiotics. If the fever and symptoms can't be managed with herbs, see a doctor.

Coughs

A cough is one of the body's defense mechanisms. It expectorates mucus and keeps the lungs clear. That being said, it is important to monitor and manage coughs to diminish the level of irritation they produce so that your body can rest, recover, and receive its needed oxygen.

When a disruptive and irritating cough is left unmanaged, many problems arise. The sleep and relaxation needed to allow the body to recover from illness is constantly interrupted. Pain is caused or made worse. Irritation is increased, causing inflammation and extreme amounts of mucus, thus interfering with breathing. In cases of croup, pneumonia, whooping cough, or RSV, the effects are not only scary but become life threatening.

When dealing with a cough, be sure you use a multidimensional approach that includes plants for internal and external use. Internally, the plants must be appropriate for the condition. It is therefore important to answer these questions. Is the cough wet and productive, or dry and irritating? Does the mucous expectorate easily, or is it sticky and immobile? Is there pain or inflammation accompanied by trouble breathing? If pain, where is it? Is there wheezing?

For external applications, I recommend aromatherapy steam inhalations, and a salve applied to the soles of the feet. The salve application is essential, as the veins in the feet run directly to the heart and respiratory tract. A salve made with antispasmodic essential oils applied to the feet help to calm a spastic cough. It is an excellent management method overnight as it can be easily reapplied without waking a child.

Aromatherapy steam inhalations are effective, for the vapors penetrate tissue directly, helping to manage a spastic cough. You may use dried plant material or essential oils. I like essential oils.

When using them, I combine the choice oils in a bottle, adding 2 drops of the formula to a heated pot of water. Turn off the heat, put your face directly over the pot, cover your head with a towel to keep the vapors in, and breath. To use a tea formula, you will basically make a tea and use this in place of the essential oil formula. The steam is hot, so be careful not to burn your face on the steam.

The essential oils I recommend for the salve and the steam are thyme, cinnamon, chamomile, lavender, and *Eucalyptus globulus*.

Tea formulas for the steam may include rosemary, cinnamon, thyme, eucalyptus, lavender, and peppermint.

Supportive Energetics for Coughs:

Anti-bacterial: garlic, usnea, goldenseal, and licorice root

Expectorants: For very wet conditions, use stimulating expectorants such as horehound, elecampane, and yerba santa. For tight and dry conditions, relaxing expectorants are necessary. Examples are thyme, licorice, garlic, grindelia, fenugreek, and plantain. Other expectorants are osha, ginger, elderberry, and good quality dark chocolate.

Immune modulators/stimulants: echinacea, ginger, and elderberry

Anti-microbial: ginger, licorice root, elderberry, thyme, yerba santa, usnea, and echinacea

Demulcents: marshmallow root, slippery elm, plantain, licorice (wet coughs do well with mullein leaf, licorice, and plantain.)

Anti-spasmodics: To control the frequency of the cough, use lobelia, wild cherry bark, mullein leaf, yerba santa, elecampane, catnip, or peppermint. When a cough does not respond to a muscular anti-spasmodic, it is time to employ skullcap. This plant, as mentioned in the *Materia medica*, calms the nerves that control the muscles of the respiratory tract, thus calming the cough.

Anti-inflammatory: licorice, chamomile, peppermint, mullein leaf, and ginger

Bronchodilators: strong black coffee (may add raw honey), American ephedra

Mucosal anti-inflammatory: hyssop, eyebright, and sage

<u>Simple Sample Cough Formulas</u>:

Below are some general examples of tea and tincture formulas for wet and dry coughs. They can and should be modified for specific illnesses.

Wet cough tea formula: 1 ounce each of the following dried plants – yerba santa or horehound, thyme, ginger, mullein leaf, and ¼ ounce of lobelia

Wet cough tincture formula: horehound, lobelia, hyssop, licorice root

Dry cough tea formula: 1 ounce each of licorice root, fresh ginger root, plantain leaf, and 1/8 ounce of lobelia. Since roots take longer, add the licorice and ginger to a quart and a half of water, bring to a boil, and then turn low. Let steep for 15 minutes. Add the other plants and let steep over low heat for 20 minutes. For severely dry coughs, use in combination with marshmallow root or slippery elm bark tea.

Dry cough tincture formula: plantain leaf, lobelia, and elecampane

General remedy for coughs: garlic and thyme tincture or syrup

Croup

Croup is an upper respiratory virus that affects mostly children aged 18 months to 9 years old. Croup is an inflammation of the larynx. While the virus lasts a mere 48-72 hours, it can be a harrowing 2-3 days for the caregiver and child, because croup can be fatal! If the larynx swells shut, air cannot pass into the lungs.

The croup cough is distinct and is the main source of consternation. It is a loud, spastic, hard cough with a seal bark at the end when air is inhaled. This bark is due to larynx swelling. The cough and inflammation are accompanied by cold symptoms such as low-grade fever (100-101 degrees), runny nose, sneezing, and, in some cases, wheezing. Inflammation and irritation is managed fairly easily during the day but worsens at night.

We have experienced croup a total of about 11 times with our children. Our oldest daughter had her first bout at 18 months and suffered through nine more bouts until she turned seven. Our youngest had it two times, but they were no less nerve wracking.

I will never forget our first time dealing with croup. Our oldest had the chicken pox, and I had taken her to the doctor to have it put in her charts to avoid immunizing. She coughed, and then came the bark. To which the doctor said, "She has croup! She needs steroids." You may already know my reply.

Croup was new to me. We went home, I made her some marshmallow root tea, began combing my old herbal texts for croup remedies and putting calls out to herbalist friends. In the end, I decided on things that made sense as opposed to being historically correct. The Eclectic doctors, for example, used an aconite and lobelia neck wrap. Our 18 month old was having nothing to do with a neck wrap, and I wasn't going with aconite.

Round one of croup was an experiment, but in round two, my medicinal wanderings became a solid plan. The end result includes therapies that came from observing the virus's effect on the body and what was needed to properly manage it according to the age of the child. Working with a stubborn and sick 18 month old has its challenges.

Here are a few notes from our process:

> Plants must lessen bronchial, trachea, and larynx irritation and inflammation.
> Employ respiratory expectorants, demulcents, and anti-spasmodics.
> Anti-viral and diaphoretic herbs are beneficial.
> Water is a great help in keeping the inflammation down with the plants.
> Mist through steam therapy and humidifiers are essential!
> Use aromatherapy to help lessen inflammation and irritation, help keep the child calm, and help manage the spastic cough. Use it on the feet, in the shower/steam therapy room, and humidifier.

> Despite the runny wet nose, the lungs are, at times, dry and irritated. Avoiding plants like ginger that are drying and too hot the first two days is essential.
> It is imperative to keep the child calm. Screaming and crying worsen inflammation, which is very bad. I will give you my favorite strategies for the task. You can also come up with your own.

Tip: If your child is prone to croup, keep these two remedies pre-made in the freezer. Make and store them separately - garlic syrup and marshmallow root infusion. I make them in September and store them through the winter, dumping any that went unused in May.

The Plant Remedies:

Herbs:

Garlic syrup: demulcent, moistening, anti-viral, expectorant, diaphoretic, warming, decongestant, anti-inflammatory

Marshmallow root tea: all the same as garlic, but cooling

Mullein leaf tea: expectorant, demulcent

Lobelia tincture: relaxing anti-spasmodic, expectorant

Licorice root tincture: demulcent, anti-viral, expectorant, diaphoretic, decongestant, anti-inflammatory

Dark chocolate: expectorant

Essential Oils: Put 1 drop of lavender, chamomile, and sweet marjoram in the steam room/shower and humidifier:

Tips: Avoid anything drying for 48-72 hours. Things in the mint family are drying, as is ginger, eyebright, and sage. After the recommended time, a weak ginger honey tea may be given (about 4 tablespoons of ginger simmered for 30 minutes in 6 cups of water). Also, add honey to anything. It, in itself, is demulcent. Don't use raw honey for children under 12 months, as it may contain botulism spores. Heating honey above 120 degrees and cooking for 15-20 minutes will kill the spores.

How to Use the Medicines:

Administer the garlic syrup and marshmallow root liberally throughout the day and overnight. I use a syringe from the store and give 2 tablespoons of marshmallow root and 1 tablespoon of the garlic syrup every hour. Of the tinctures: lobelia, 1-2 drops 4 times, and 1-2 times overnight; licorice root, 5-10 drops 4 times daily, and 1-2 times overnight.

Essential oils should be used in the humidifier throughout the day and night; add 1-2 drops of each oil listed above. Add more every 2-3 hours.

Overnight

When your child wakes up coughing and barking, bring them to the bathroom and shut the door. Turn the shower on hot, add a drop of each essential oil to the tub, and let the scent and steam fill the room. Encourage breathing. You will be in this spot for 10-15 minutes, so you may want to bring a blanket. This is where calming methods come in handy, which is in the section below.

Once out of the bathroom and back in bed, your child should take some of the marshmallow root infusion and have a bit of water. If anti-spasmodics are needed, give the lobelia and licorice tincture.

A child with croup may wake up often overnight. Keep with the schedule above when they do.

Calming Methods

Distraction will engage the mind, and it is your best friend. From talking to counting, storytelling to singing, this is the time to use your awesome parenting skills. And it won't be easy. You might be afraid, exhausted, and stressed.

When will you use these methods? Anytime your child is upset. Remember, crying and screaming fuel inflammation, which is to be avoided.

Story telling is an excellent way to calm. You can make up stories about the plants you are using, weave a fairy tale, or tell childhood stories about yourself or other relatives. The bathroom with the door shut and the shower running is a great place for stories. One can easily be transported by the sound of water falling into the tub and the scented air. You can even use the presence of the two as props to begin your tale, incorporating your return to bed as the ending.

Other tools you can use to augment your story are counting and drawing. Allow bathroom tiles, bathtub toys, toes and fingers to become counting props. Or draw little pictures to illustrate your tale. Sometimes, your child will even join in.

Singing songs is another balm for calm. Rock your wee one while you sing. Sing songs you know, or make them up!

Earaches

Earaches may be caused by an infection, fluid, or swelling in the ear, sinuses, or throat. Infection in the outer ear is called *otitis extrena*. It may be caused by an object, boil, or scratching of the canal.

A middle ear infection, *otitis media*, occurs in the part of the ear directly behind the eardrum. These accompany upper respiratory infections.

Things to do if ear pain is present:

- Stay upright and wrap the neck in warm compresses or a heating pad. Do this several times daily.
- Use a warm compress of castor or olive oil with oils of lavender and rosemary rubbed on the neck and around the outside of the ear.
- I recommend eardrops made with olive oil infused mullein flower, St. John's wort, and garlic with a few drops of goldenseal glycerin. According to Mary Bove, ND, glycerin is specific for absorbing excess water and fluid. You can use equal parts of the oils. Mix the ingredients and warm the drops to body temperature. Using cold drops will cause extreme pain. Put about 2-4 drops into the ear, and insert cotton to contain it.
  Warning: Never use ear drops if the eardrum is ruptured (caused by middle ear infection; discharge either bloody or pussy, buzzing in the ear, and a sharp pain that is decreased quickly after).

- Address complicating factors such as sore throat or sinus congestion for relief.
- Energetics and herbs to use for ear congestion are decongestant, lymphatic herbs, and anti-microbial/bacterial.

Tincture formula for ear pain with sinus congestion: 5 ml of cayenne, 5 ml horseradish, 10 ml calendula, 10 ml of echinacea. Adults take 35 drops 4-6 times daily until symptoms retreat. Children ages 5-12 take 15-20 drops 4-6 times daily until better. Also consider adding strong cups of ginger tea with honey.

Herbs to consider: cleavers, calendula, cayenne, goldenseal, echinacea, ginger, and usnea

Fevers (Are Fearless)

The fever is our body's answer to illness. It's unyielding in its power and fearlessness. Yet the occurrence of a fever can ignite fear in the sufferer or care giver, especially if it reaches great heights.

For myself, I had experience successfully dealing with fevers at my herb store. The plants specific for them I knew well, so I imagined having no problem managing fevers in my own children. But when my first daughter's fevers began to reach 105+, I was shaken. For the first time in my life, I feared the fever and my ability to assist it naturally.

One day, as my daughter's fever spiked to 105, and no herb, drug, or drink would break it, I heard this little voice whisper, "*Verbena hastata*" (common name blue vervain). I knew it was a diaphoretic but had never tried it on her fevers before. I prepared 20 drops of the bitter tincture in a teaspoon of water. She took it, and it worked!

This experience inspired me to begin thinking differently about fevers. I started making note of symptom pictures, realizing that there were different kinds of fevers with a variety of forces that drove them. I also considered the idea of functional and dysfunctional heat in the body when infection is present and applied plants according to taste for fever management.

My research also unearthed historical treatment methods beyond drinking teas and taking tinctures. For example, in old literature I found reference to herbal or vinegar footbaths, and, in Anthroposophical books, discovered soaking socks in lemon.

I still obsess about my oldest daughter's fevers, for her nature is to run an extremely high temperature when ill. But each time they rise, I'm reminded that her fevers presence inspired me to consider new ideas, which I hope to illustrate here.

Physiology of a Fever:

The hypothalamus sits at the base of the brain. One of its jobs is to control body temperature. When the body perceives an illness, it triggers a chemical message to be sent through the blood stream to the hypothalamus. This message informs the hypothalamus that a pathogen, either viral or bacterial, is attempting to proliferate. Because our body knows that such invaders are temperature sensitive, the thermostat is turned up as the battle for health begins.

There are two popular terms used to describe the stage of a fever. One is *spike*, and the other is *break*. Each stage is accompanied by its own set of symptoms, which may vary per person.

When the core temperature begins to rise, or spike, metabolic activity is increased. The blood circulates from the periphery to the interior. The sufferer may not necessarily feel hot to touch despite the rise in temperature. If the temperature spikes above 102, sweat may be suppressed, leaving the skin to feel dry and warm. A temperature spike may also be characterized by shivering, with complaints of being cold. You can see tension on the face, and one may feel jittery and unable to relax due to constriction in the nervous system. Some may become sensitive to light and sound, and their eyes may burn.

When the fever breaks, blood mobilizes out to the periphery. The pores of the skin may be red and dilated. One will feel hot and begin to perspire. Facial expression and body posture will relax, which will show in the eyes. It is as if a steam valve has been released, and the body sighs in relief.

Energetics to consider for fever treatment are:

- Diaphoretics (either stimulating, or relaxing)
- Anti-inflammatory
- Anti-microbial
- Anti-bacterial

As we go through treatment plans for each type of fever, we'll plug in where the energetics fit.

Treatment plan for a low-grade fever:

A low-grade fever for a child or adult is 99-101 degrees. It will typically accompany a viral infection. The spikes and breaks will occur on a small scale and are far less dramatic than those of the high fevers.

There are times when someone with excess heat exposure, cancer, or autoimmune disease might run a low-grade fever. I will be discussing treatment plans for those associated with acute infections.

Quick list of symptoms:

- Low-grade fever with viral infection
- Spikes that don't go above 101.9 degrees
- Body is hot and sweats easily
- Chills are not debilitating
- Fever manages well with fluids and hot teas

Sample Treatment Formulas:

Low-grade fevers manage well with little interference and respond to simple teas and increased fluid intake. A most effective plant approach should include something to warm the circulatory system, thereby stimulating the body's ability to fight infection, for it is believed, and rightly so, that a cold/weak internal climate is one reason people fall prey to acute illness.

Examples of tea formulas:

General tea: 1-2 teaspoons each of chamomile, yarrow, lavender and catnip (or linden – see diaphoretic definition for specifics).

Warming tea: 2 teaspoons holy basil, ½ teaspoon of cardamom, 2 teaspoons yarrow, 1 teaspoon grated ginger, 1-2 teaspoons honey; steep 10 minutes.

Flu tea: 2 teaspoons yarrow, 1 teaspoon elder flower, 2 teaspoons fresh grated ginger rhizome, 1 teaspoon honey; steep 10 minutes.

Hot toddy: 2 tablespoons of grated ginger, juice of 1 fresh lemon, 8 ounces hot water, and honey to taste; steep 10 minutes. Drink as hot as tolerated.

Tinctures are not usually necessary for the low-grade fever, but I find them excellent for nighttime management or for other symptoms of an illness. If support is needed for other symptoms, please refer to their appropriate section. General tincture formulas for the low-grade fever are as follows.

Examples of tincture formulas:

Equal parts of *Angelica archangelica*, calendula, ginger, and yarrow.

Equal parts of turmeric, calendula, yarrow, catnip (or linden).

My favorite low-grade fever remedy is a hot toddy and a strong cup of yarrow tea with honey.

My favorite tincture is angelica, calendula, ginger, and yarrow.

Illustration of a treatment plan for low-grade fever with depressed immunity:

This low-grade fever is similar in nature to the one first mentioned, lacking the drama of a high fever in spikes and dips. But the root of this low fever is different. It stems from an acute illness that has difficulty being fought, will be long lasting, and have a tendency to recur. I call this low-grade fever with depressed immunity. The depression is caused by excess cold in the system.

One of my favorite examples of this type of infection comes from an old student. She came to me after class complaining of a recurrent bacterial infection that would not respond to plants or allopathic medications. It was accompanied by a chronic low-grade fever. I listened while she explained a condition that she believed was hot and needed cooling due to the fact that she felt prickly heat where the infection was located.

I pointed out that what she had described to me was a condition of coldness with a depressed immune system, despite the hot and prickly nature. Her chronic acute infection and low-grade fever were signs that her immune system would not be stimulated and that she should consider warming agents to do so.

She changed her plan to one of warming the immune system and the area affected. I gave her some yerba mansa root, and she decided to try turmeric. The infection responded beautifully and was gone in a few days time.

Quick list of symptoms:

- Low-grade fever with recurring infection despite treatment (viral or bacterial).
- Sufferer is exhausted but still able to work.
- May have hot feelings in localized areas (throat, vagina, eyes, lungs), but the body is unable to efficiently fight the infection.

Recommended treatment plan:

Plants that warm and stimulate are essential allies here. In my opinion, the depressed fever is no place for acrid bitters or relaxants, unless someone needs them to get to sleep at night. Relaxation comes when the body is effectively functioning. In this case, that involves plants that warm the blood and stimulate.

Examples of tea:

Hot toddy (ginger, lemon, honey in hot water; see instructions for making under low-grade fever)

Teas of holy basil, elderflower, ginger, yarrow

Tinctures:

Tincture formulas should be dependent on symptom picture and illness. Be sure to include lymphatics that act as immune tonics in your formula and plants that warm the blood to stimulate immunity.

Examples of diaphoretic plants to consider in tincture form for depressed immunity: *Angelica archangelica*, calendula, holy basil, cardamom, echinacea, elderflower, licorice, usnea, and turmeric.

Treatment plan for a high fever:

High fevers in children can run 102-106, and for adults, 102-104. A temperature of 104-106 in an adult is dangerous. From my perspective, high fevers are a result of the blood being trapped at the core of the body, constricting the nervous, immune, and circulatory systems. The bound circulatory system cannot disperse blood out, and, in some cases, will also immobilize the immune system. Perspiration is scant, and the nervous system becomes over stimulated, resulting in a very high fever.

While fevers of this nature generally result from bacterial infections, there are some strains of the flu and other viruses that can cause them. I have also found that some children are simply prone to high fevers.

Quick list of symptoms:

- Temperature, high and rising, seems stuck
- Inability to relax, agitated and nervous
- Severe chills with hot head and cold feet
- Bodily shakes and tremors
- Sometimes joint pain
- Skin warm and dry
- Little or no ability to perspire
- Burning eyes and/or bloodshot eyes
- Sensitive to light and sound
- In some cases, won't respond to acetaminophen or Motrin
- Breaks in temperature yield only a slight and temporary decrease

Recommended treatment plan:

The high fever is rooted in the nervous system, thereby defining a need for the diaphoretics that are relaxing. These plants release stuck tension and heat from the nervous system without further stimulating and heating the already boiling blood. Their bitterness (acrid bitter, to be taste descriptive) brings on a shiver once it hits the tongue.

Plants in this category are blue vervain, catnip, linden blossom, and yarrow. Yarrow is not as acrid, but it complements the others very well, and I feel it is specifically indicated for high fevers with the flu. If there is a complete inability to sweat, catnip is necessary.

Because the impetus of this fever is also infection, acrid bitters must be balanced with aromatic/pungents that are anti-infective. Consider plants like turmeric, *Angelica archangelica*, usnea, or calendula, which won't heat the blood too much, but will be supportive. Pick your aromatic/pungent plant that will compliment your acrid relaxing diaphoretic based on symptom pictures and the infection.

I recommend using teas and tinctures throughout the day. Footbaths and warm socks soaked in lemon or tea will also help fever management immensely (instructions will be given).

Examples of tea and tincture formulas:

Tea: equal parts chamomile, yarrow, catnip (or linden blossom)
Supportive tincture: blue vervain, calendula, catnip (or linden blossom), ginger

Tea: yarrow, catnip (linden blossom), holy basil
Supportive tincture: *Angelica archangelica*, blue vervain, licorice, yarrow

Tea: yarrow, peppermint, catnip, chamomile
Supportive tincture: blue vervain, catnip, ginger, turmeric

Dangers of high fevers:

High fevers are hazardous for many reasons. Not only can the heat cause brain damage in all individuals, but it can also incite seizures in children. Please employ caution when treating them and follow these guidelines recommended by the Mayo Health Clinic and Mary Bove, N.D.

It is time to consult with your doctor or to seek emergency care when:

- The fever lasts longer than three days, for there may be a bacterial infection
- There is confusion or lethargy with inability to communicate
- Body twitching
- Listlessness with vomiting and headaches
- It is a child under six months

Symptoms which may complicate fever management:

Bacterial infections: If a high fever lasts for more than 3-5 days and takes constant maintenance, and if symptoms are worsening, please seek the advice of a trained professional. There are instances where a bacterial infection is present. If the bacteria are not responding quickly enough to herbs, an antibiotic may be necessary.

Constipation: This can be a sign that there is too much dryness. Any blocked channel of elimination (urinary, colon, skin, respiratory) makes fever management difficult. Try drinking tea infusions of either dandelion root or marshmallow root. (Refer to the *Materia medica* for medicine making instructions.) Enemas may also be helpful.

Inability to sweat: Sweating is how the body cools itself. When a sweat cannot be broken, heat builds. Drink a fresh ginger root tea as hot as possible, or drink catnip and yarrow tea. A foot bath in ginger or lemon, or socks soaked in lemon are effective as well. (See instructions in the next section.)

Vomiting and/or fluid loss: A fever with stomachache or vomiting can be a difficult combination. With this symptom combination, tinctures for fever management are essential. You may use one or a combination of two of the following: yarrow, blue vervain, peppermint, and chamomile. They are well tolerated and can help manage vomiting. If intestinal cramps are debilitating, try the homeopathic magnesia phosphorica. Holding down fluids may be impossible, but I learned from Mary Bove, N.D. that small amounts of fluid are effective. Have the person drink 1 teaspoon-1 tablespoon of an electrolyte fluid every 20 minutes until more can be held down. I use Emergen-C or a weak dilutions of peppermint, yarrow, or chamomile tea with a little raw honey added.

Inability to consume enough fluid: Some kids can't stand to drink when they are ill. It's important to have a strategy when this occurs. Here are mine:

- A game called "Cheers Sip." You need 2 cups of fluid (one for you and one for them) and a dice. Roll the dice and you both say "Cheers Sip," and drink the number of sips the dice tells you. Do this about every 20 minutes to keep fluid intake up. Keep playing until your child is more willing to drink on their own.
- Another tool I like to use is a syringe. You can get them at drug stores. I give 2 tablespoons every 15-20 minutes.
- Purchase straws. I don't condone the use of them often for they are wasteful. But when a child is coughing, suffering from a stuffy nose or tired, sipping is difficult. Straws make drinking easier, and the fun colors they come in brighten the day.
- When kids tire of fluid consumption switch to tinctures. If their fever is really high, try the footbaths and soaked socks in the following section.

Foot Bath Teas

My love and interest in footbaths began after I read the book *Of Plants and People*, by Maurice *Mességué*. He successfully treated all maladies, both chronic and acute, with herb hand

and foot baths. After experiencing my own personal success treating heat exposure with footbaths, I was inspired to try them on fevers, and was excited by the success. There were times a 104 temperature would fall to 100 within minutes of the feet hitting the water. While it wasn't the remedy that always broke the fever, it helped to manage the temperature while the teas and tinctures did their work.

Instructions for footbath:

1. Choose the tea of your choice based on your symptoms. My favorites are yarrow (excellent in general), catnip (if trouble sweating), linden blossom (if the skin is hot and moist), and ginger (if cold/depressed).
2. Steep 3 tablespoons of herb in 2 cups of hot water for 10 minutes. Add it to a basin with enough warm water to cover the feet. At this point, 2 drops of lavender essential oil may also be added.
3. Soak for about 20 minutes.
4. Repeat as needed throughout the day.

Lemon Socks

Lemon socks are an effective way to reduce a fever. They pull heat from the head down to the feet and disperse it throughout the body. When the heat is moved, it becomes an active tool for fighting infection, and the temperature drops. You can also use diaphoretic teas such as yarrow and linden flower, and some people use vinegar.

Fevers tend to spike before bed. So this is the routine I follow. I give my kids a few ounces of fever tea and a good dose of tincture (about 30 drops of a formula in a teaspoon of warm water). I then put warm lemon socks on their feet for 20 minutes while they fall asleep and follow with another tincture dose an hour later.

To prepare the socks:

Take one lemon, juice it, add it to ¼ cup of hot water. Soak cotton socks in the water, ring them, let them cool slightly, and put them on the feet. Next, cover the feet with wool socks, and cover the body to keep it warm. Allow the socks to remain on for 20 minutes.

Feeling incapable? While it is good to avoid drugs, the learning curve can sometimes be steep, especially when a bacterial infection is present. You haven't failed if you need to reach for something other than plant or alternative medicines.

Flu

Symptoms: bone chills, fever up to 105, headache, sore throat, cough, diarrhea, and vomiting in children with abdominal cramping, extreme fatigue, eyes feel as if they are burning and stinging.

Just as with the common cold, heat the body to get natural defenses up. A strong cup of hot ginger tea with honey is great for this.

Tincture formula: yarrow, elderberry, cardamom, echinacea, licorice root, add boneset for bone chilling pain

For extreme diarrhea: It's best to let it run its course. But when a break is needed, drink raspberry leaf tea. We often use this for overnights when getting rest is most important.

Tea: ginger, linden blossom, yarrow

Vomiting: Take Emergen-C or herbal tincture mix by the tablespoon full every 20 minutes until able to hold more down.

Homeopathic: For abdominal cramping, use magnesia phosphorica.

Aromatherapy: thyme, *Eucalyptus globulus* or *radiata*, geranium, oregano, frankincense, and cinnamon

Headaches

Headaches associated with respiratory infections can be the result of sinus congestion, fever, or simply general inflammation.

Herbs and essential oils with the following supportive energetics should be considered: nervine, analgesic, anti-inflammatory, and decongestant.

For headaches with sinus congestion, I recommend a steam inhalation with peppermint and chamomile teas, and also an aromatherapy formula of decongestants and anti-inflammatory plants applied to the forehead, at the temples, and back of the neck.

This should be prepared as a 1% dilution (6 drops of pure essential oil in 1 ounce of carrier oil). A drop or two of essential oil can also be used in a steam inhalation.

Sample formulas:

Worry Wart Headache Relief Tea: peppermint, chamomile, skullcap, and yarrow. If something warming is needed, add ginger.

Noggin Numbing Aromatherapy Formula: Essential oils of lavender, eucalyptus, peppermint, and yarrow. Add 3 drops of yarrow, 3 drops of lavender, 2 drops of eucalyptus, and 1 drop of peppermint to a ½ ounce of carrier oil. Apply at temples every 15 minutes and inhale deeply until desired result is achieved. I also recommend adding clove pure essential oil if something warming is needed.

Headache Tincture: blue vervain, skullcap, peppermint, and yarrow. Take 35 drops every 30-45 minutes as needed until the headache subsides.

Sinus Tincture: horseradish and elecampane

Sedatives

When some are faced with an illness, they naturally become exhausted and rest easily. There are also those who become agitated and have trouble relaxing. I consider agitation an official symptom that needs intervention, for when we rest, we heal.

Because agitation is also a symptom of high fever, or a fever that is spiking, check the temperature. Using a nervine tonic, such as blue vervain, for a high or spiking fever can decrease agitation. Also, keep the T.V. turned off in instances of agitation as it can often aggravate and make the individual more nervous.

Herb teas are a great way to calm and sedate while hydrating. I always add a bit of raw honey, which helps maintain electrolytes and is slightly calming. Teas to consider: chamomile, lavender, linden blossom, lemon balm, and yarrow.

Tinctures pack a powerful punch as well. Blue vervain, passionflower, and catnip are all diaphoretic and sedative.

Essential oils can not only help fight infection, but can also help the ill and infirmed relax. Oils that may be supportive therapy are clary sage, lavender, lemongrass, vetiver, or sweet mandarin.

Methods of application may include one or all of the following:

- A formula of a 3% dilution to be applied 2-3 times daily and at bedtime to the feet. You may remember that the veins in the feet run directly to the heart and respiratory tract, treating agitation, sleeplessness, and lower respiratory infections very well.
- An Epsom salt bath in lavender and lemongrass (add about a teaspoon of essential oils per cup of salt).
- Use a few drops of one or more of the essential oils in a cold air humidifier throughout the day for relaxation.
- Try a few drops of one of the essential oils on a warm wet washcloth applied to the forehead or neck. Inhale deeply.

Sinus Congestion and Sinusitis

Sinus congestion and inflammation can be a symptom of sinusitis, which is inflammation and infection of the sinuses. Symptoms include headache, postnasal drip, yellow-green mucus, fever, cough, and sore throat. It can cause an earache, toothache, and pain and swelling of the face.

Formulas should include plants according to symptoms:

Tincture: barberry, echinacea, licorice root, fenugreek, or horseradish (if something stronger is needed)

Decongestants (to help decrease swelling and stuffiness): horseradish, cayenne, ginger, and elderberry
- Plants specific for green discharge: elecampane and usnea
- Plants specific for yellow discharge: elecampane and goldenseal
- Clear very wet secretions: sage and raspberry leaf
- Lymphatics: echinacea, calendula, or cleavers
- Warm to thin fluid: cayenne, ginger and garlic

Tincture sample formulas: cayenne, elecampane, horseradish, calendula; or echinacea, elecampane, ginger

Teas to think about: ginger, peppermint, plantain, or sage

Aromatherapy can be a friend for those suffering from sinus congestion. The vapors penetrate the tissue directly, which speeds healing and lessens the risk of infection going deeper or mutating. You may use dried plant material or essential oils.

Methods of Application:

Make an herbal steam sauna for your face. Take a bowl of heated water, not so hot that you asphyxiate yourself with aroma, but hot enough to create steam. Add 5 drops total of a combination of essential oils. Make a tent with a towel over your head and inhale for about 5 minutes. Do this three times daily. Essential oils I recommend are thyme, cinnamon, chamomile, lavender, *Eucalyptus globulus*, and rosemary.

Take a hot bath with essential oils in Epsom salts.

Apply a salve containing the chosen oils to the neck and wrap in a warm wet towel with a dry one over it to help contain the heat. This is not as direct a method as the others, but still mildly effective.

I also like to heat a small pot of water, turn off the fire, and add the oils. They diffuse into the air and help relieve sinus congestion

Sore Throat

Sore throats respond to anti-inflammatories, astringents, and/or to demulcents. At times, all that is needed is a nice spoonful of raw honey. When a sore throat is caused by postnasal drip or a cough, one must deal with those issues as well.

General tinctures: red root (only if really wet), echinacea, licorice root, osha, and sage

Soothing teas: marshmallow root, chamomile, slippery elm, fenugreek, sage

Profuse clear secretions with sore throat: sage or raspberry leaf tea with raw honey

Stomach Virus

The approach with stomach viruses is to let them run their course, using plant therapies to help manage symptoms and discomfort and to help avoid dehydration.

Symptoms that may arise are diarrhea, severe cramping, low-grade fever, vomiting, nausea, and headaches.

With diarrhea, manage it with teas throughout the day (see below). When it's time to sleep, I get out the raspberry leaf with catnip tincture. If you have a high fever, add yarrow tincture. Kids get about 15-20 drops 2 times before bed, while adults get closer to 35 drops.

Vomiting makes managing some symptoms, such as fever or cramping, difficult. I recommend using tinctures for the fever in this case, with the dehydration tip below. Try something as simple as yarrow with blue vervain. Also, there is a homeopathic that works beautifully for cramping. It's magnesia phosphorica, potency 6 cc. Take 5 pellets every 15 minutes until cramps are relieved. Once teas are tolerated, I usually do one plant or maybe two plants at a time.

Dehydration is often a danger with stomach viruses. There are times when it seems that no fluid is tolerated. But I learned from a wonderful N.D. named Mary Bove that giving a teaspoon or tablespoon of fluid every 30-60 minutes is all it takes to make a difference. I recommend alternating between Emergen-C for electrolyte loss and teas of peppermint and raspberry leaf with honey. Avoid cold water, as it can cause severe cramping.

Some herbs to use:

Tincture: yarrow, chamomile, catnip, blue vervain, and bee balm (my favorites)

Teas: yarrow, chamomile, licorice, cardamom, raspberry leaf, and marshmallow root for burning or irritation

Homeopathic: magnesia phosphorica 6 cc. for cramping is much better tolerated when vomiting than herbs for cramping.

<u>Symptoms with herbal suggestions</u>:

Fever: tincture of catnip, blue vervain, yarrow, bee balm; teas of yarrow, licorice

Diarrhea: tincture of yarrow, raspberry leaf, peppermint; teas of yarrow, raspberry leaf, black tea

Vomiting: tincture of blue vervain, bee balm, peppermint, anise hyssop; teas of peppermint, bee balm, anise hyssop

Nausea: tincture of peppermint, blue vervain, bee balm, ginger; teas of peppermint, bee balm, ginger

Abdominal cramping: peppermint tea, homeopathic magnesia phosphorica 6 cc.

Dehydration: teas with honey, Emergen-C

Swollen Lymph Nodes/Glands

Swollen lymph nodes can pop up with streptococcal pharyngitis (strep throat). But they can also be a direct result of our body fighting a simple viral infection.

Lymphatic herbs can be extremely effective at reducing swelling and supporting the immune system. A few that I love to use are cleavers, echinacea, red root, calendula, and small amounts of poke root. Calendula and echinacea are also immune potentiating. The others are essential in supporting lymphatic circulation to decrease fluid buildup.

Essential oil neck rub for swollen glands/lymphatic swelling: 2 drops each of the following in a carrier oil: bay laurel, vetiver, frankincense. Apply to lymph nodes on the neck or anywhere there is lymphatic swelling. Continue use until the swelling recedes.

A salt-water gargle also reduces tonsil swelling almost immediately. The salt washing over the swollen tonsils inspires them to purge the contents. Salt is also anti-bacterial and anti-microbial. This needs to be done repeatedly to be effective. I have seen tonsils nearly swollen together from a strep infection shrink by half.

General tincture formula for swollen glands: 11 ml of calendula, 11 ml of cleavers, and 3 ml of poke root

Strep support tincture: 10 ml calendula, 10 ml echinacea, 10 ml cleavers, 5 ml poke root; can be used with an antibiotic; adults take 35 drops 3-4 times daily for 2 weeks; children age 5-12 take 15 drops 3-4 times daily for 2 weeks. For recurrent strep in children, take 5-10 drops 2-3 times daily for 3-6 months.

Mononucleosis

Lymphatic, spleen, and liver swelling are of main concern here. A specific herb for mono spleen swelling is red root (*Ceanothus americanus*). In fact, if it's the only or one of a few plants you take for mono, please take this one. If you are interested in a tincture formula for mono, here is one good example. Equal parts echinacea, calendula, red root, dandelion root, and grindelia. Take 15-35 drops of this formula 3-4 times daily for 10 days. After that, continue with a tincture of equal parts red root, echinacea, and milk thistle. Take 5-15 drops 3-4 times daily for about a month.

Chapter Wrap-up

Things to Remember:

- Dosages are not the same for everyone. Experiment to find your therapeutic dose.
- Formulas are suggestions. You can use them, but getting specific to you is beneficial.
- Be sure to study the plants you would like to use. Refer to the *Materia medica* or other resources. Choose the ones that fit you and your symptoms the best.
- Give what you've chosen time to work.
- Remember to drink a healthy amount of water!
- If acute infections plague you frequently, please find a good herbalist who can help you with a long-term solution.

Chapter 9

Insomnia and Stress; Tincture and Essential Oil Formulas to Induce Sleep

Rosa's Story

I met Rosa when we lived in New Mexico. A descendant of Mayan farmers, she was the quintessential abuela (grandmother). She was warm and soft, with a physical sturdiness, rooted nature, and strong sense of self that made one feel at ease when near her.

She and her husband had moved to the United States to farm. And despite being in their 70's, were a weekly fixture at the local farmer's market. Their crops were prominently displayed in classic New Mexico style, with chili pepper ristras hanging from the sides of their tent and a colorful array of seasonal vegetables, fruits, and gourds.

My husband and I developed a close bond with Rosa. Whenever she saw us coming with our new baby, she was effusive, treating us more like family than customers. As we shopped, she would coo over the baby, while casually tucking extra ears of corn, potatoes, or cilantro into our bag.

It wasn't long before Rosa discovered I was an herbalist and asked for help dealing with a few health problems. As it turned out, she had more than a few, accompanied by an extensive health history, which included surviving two bouts of cancer, heart disease, and open heart surgery.

Rosa's current complaints were: red patches of itchy dry skin on her arms, arthritis, mild high blood pressure, anxiety with depression and insomnia, digestive distress with acid reflux, and anemia.

I began with what seemed like the simplest place, because it involved a perfect plant that Rosa grew in copious amounts – chamomile!

Chamomile is an antacid, nervine tonic, anti-anxiety, demulcent, anti-inflammatory, and is excellent for insomnia. Rosa was to drink three cups of tea between meals and wash her arms in a tea bath. To support the work of her body healing and improve her digestive health, Rosa also agreed to eat less cheese. Her diet was excellent, otherwise. The protocol worked beautifully, improving her health and relieving many of her symptoms in a few weeks time.

I observed how she responded to the chamomile and decided to add an anti-inflammatory salve made with essential oils of ginger, rosemary, eucalyptus, and lavender with arnica infused oil for her joint pain, and a tincture of yellow dock root, burdock root, and red root (15 drops before meals, three times daily) to improve digestion, assimilation, swelling in the villa of the small intestine, and joint inflammation. She responded beautifully to the salve, and the tincture formula.

Insomnia

The constantly suffering insomniac wakes to many dawns of exhaustion. This exhaustion disables the body's ability to do important tasks and makes insomnia a precursor for more serious health problems, from digestive distress to anxiety. But it doesn't stop there.

- The immune system and body's ability to heal kicks in as we sleep. When we don't rest, we are more prone to acute and chronic illness, and take longer to recover.
- Appropriate rest and relaxation gives our adrenals and nervous system a break, preparing us to more capably deal with stress and be more emotionally balanced.
- Insomnia can lead to anxiety, depression, and emotional distress, further affecting the heart and digestive organs.

When working with clients, sleeplessness is one of the first problems I address. It can be a multilayered process, involving aromatherapy and internal use of plant medicines, dietary modification, and lifestyle adjustments. Our plan will also involve how to improve one's ability to deal with stress, both physically and emotionally.

Stress

Stress is a byproduct of being a living human being. It is a natural part of the vital life force. Stress can motivate us to complete a project and inspire us to focus. But it can also be a nuisance, distracting and undermining our work, as well as drastically destabilizing our mental and physical health. From insomnia and anxiety, to digestive disorders and depressed immunity, stress hits us at our weakest point.

Relieving and managing stress is one of the most important things we can do for our health. Not only can it increase our quality of life, but the supportive tools we employ to alleviate it can alter how we deal with and react to stress in the future. This allows us to become more adaptable in stressful situations, making life's woes more bearable.

The process of learning to live with and lessen the effects of stress does not happen without a bit of effort. And there is an abundance of advice on the subject. Lifestyle changes are especially popular. The counsel is sound and often includes sensible things, such as the following:

1. Get proper sleep.
2. Eat a whole foods, low processed sugar diet with no soda and low caffeine.
3. Drink plenty of water.
4. Get regular exercise.
5. Involve yourself in enjoyable activities that make you feel good - meditation, yoga, art, writing or music, for example.

There are times, however, when change is not enough. Our reaction to stress is perpetuated by our body's inability to break an internal cycle, and our life's inability to give us a break. Help is needed to restore balance and redirect energy. And plant medicines can be very effective here, especially in the way of nervine tonics.

What is a Nervine Tonic?

Tonics, as I mentioned in Chapter 1, nourish, tone, and retrain the body. Their effects can be felt immediately, but the best results are seen when taken over a long period of time, for they work slowly to inspire deep and long standing changes internally.

A tonic coaxes the organ to remember balance and function by one or more of the following actions: relaxing, stimulating, moistening to soften, drying to harden, heating to disperse energy, or cooling to restrain it. They have the capacity to invigorate function when an organ system is deficient or under-functioning, or reduce activity when it is excessive.

Nervine tonics have many of these effects on the nervous system. For this reason, their use in insomnia is essential. They help improve a person's stress response and symptoms of that response long term. But they don't stop there. They also have an affinity for other organ systems with secondary effects that support multiple processes of the body.

For example, it is known that stress can cause digestive distress. And many herbs that calm the nervous system also influence digestion. Chamomile is one. It calms the nervous system, is anti-inflammatory, demulcent (soothing irritated tissues), carminative (dispelling gas in the intestinal tract), and is antacid. Chamomile is also slightly bitter, stimulating bile release from the liver to support digestion and assimilation of nutrients. Its anti-inflammatory properties also assist the colonization of healthy bowel flora in the large intestine.

Nervines and other plant medicines may be magical enchantments, but they won't make everything perfect. And their job is not to change us or make everything we are experiencing go away. They do slow our reaction to the world around us down from a run to a walk, making uncomfortable and unbearable feelings more manageable. With this change in tempo, our head and heart become synchronized, allowing our whole body to align with a healthier circadian rhythm over time.

Picking Your Nervine Tonic

Choosing the right nervine tonic is a matter of taking aspects of health and personality into account. And while someone trained in herbalism might consider many things when recommending plants, picking your own is often as simple as answering a few questions and reading about a few plants. Here are some questions to consider.

1. What are your symptoms when stressed?
2. Do you suffer from anxiety, insomnia, acute reoccurring illness, or digestive distress?
3. Are you a hot head who needs something cooling to pull heat down, or something warming to relax and break through cold blockages?

It's impossible to talk about insomnia without talking about stress. The two are inseparable. Now, let's look at how to put some of those tinctures you have made and essential oils you've accumulated to work.

Some Great Nervines To Consider

- Catnip
- Linden
- Milky oat seed
- Motherwort
- Passionflower
- Skullcap
- St. John's wort

Further descriptions can be found in Chapter 11.

Aromatherapy Vs. Tincture

There are specific reasons I would choose aromatherapy over a tincture. For one, aromatherapy helps set the mind and body in a relaxed direction quickly, for it has a direct effect on chemical firings in the brain. And, more importantly, because it's applied topically, I can avoid herb drug interactions or simplify how many plants are being taken internally.

Note: You'll notice I said tincture above and not tea. I avoid teas when trying to get someone to sleep. I don't want my client disrupting their sleep cycle to visit the bathroom.

Aromatherapy for Insomnia

The Essential Oils

Sedative: rose, spikenard, sweet mandarin, clary sage, chamomile

Balancing (with some sedative effects): lavender, geranium, vetiver, and frankincense

Sample Formulas and the Nightly Application Process

Applications for sedation should be administered through the feet, over the heart, and on the neck. The veins in the feet run directly to the heart and respiratory tract, bypassing the liver and delivering medicine right to the source.

I recommend application 20-30 minutes before bed. I also recommend healing baths with an oil or bath salt formula for insomnia. Dilutions: Adults use 7 drops of essential oil total in 1 ounce of carrier oil. Kids ages 4-10 use 5 drops of essential oil total in 1 ounce of carrier oil.

Sample Insomnia Formulas

- Lavender, lemongrass
- Sweet mandarin, frankincense
- Lavender, clary sage
- Chamomile, lemongrass, lavender
- Spikenard, frankincense, sweet mandarin
- Rosewood, spikenard, and sweet mandarin

Insomnia in Kids and the Elderly

Kids and the elderly find scent comforting. It can improve grumpy exhausted moods and increase the quality of sleep, thereby improving mood the next day. They often respond to simple therapies, such as lavender pillows or a drop of lavender, lemongrass, or sweet mandarin pure essential oil near their bed.

When speaking to hospitals and hospice groups, I suggest putting a drop of essential oil on a cotton ball, and placing the ball inside the pillowcase. It works great in institutional and assisted living situations, because it's an effective, easy, and inexpensive solution.

Another great application method is the foot rub, as mentioned above. Add a few drops of one or two different essential oils to a salve or lotion base, and massage into the feet. Foot rubs can be a great bedtime bonding tool, facilitating relaxation and a chance to chat about the day.

Sample Tincture Formulas for Insomnia

Insomnia with cold and depressed immune function, prone to acute infections: equal parts tincture of lavender, motherwort, passionflower; 35-70 drops 30 minutes before bed.

Insomnia with anxiety and heat rising to the head: equal parts tincture of passionflower, motherwort, and hawthorn; 35-70 drops 30 minutes before bed.

Insomnia with heart palpitations and high blood pressure: motherwort, hawthorn, fresh milky oat: 20-35 drops 30 minutes before bed

Insomnia that stems from an excessive use of stimulants, leading to an inability to sleep and exhaustion during the day: Retraining the rhythm of the body is important. I use a daytime and nighttime formula to do this.

Daytime tincture: equal parts of Siberian ginseng, holy basil, and milky oat tincture; 10-20 drops 3-4 times daily. Cease use of this tincture after 4 pm.

Nighttime tincture: motherwort, milky oats, passionflower; 35-70 drops 30 minutes before bed.

Note: I have successfully used this approach with former drug addicts. They must be off drugs and have gone through withdrawal. Others who benefit from this approach are weaning mothers and those who do overnight care for the elderly and infirmed.

A Few of My Favorite Formulas:

- Hawthorn, passionflower, motherwort
- Blue vervain, skullcap, passionflower
- Oats, skullcap, California poppy

What If You Wake Up?

There are those who wake up naturally as they learn to re-balance sleep cycles. I recommend taking another 35 drops of tincture or reapplying the aromatherapy formula and going back to bed.

Suggestions for Lifestyle Modification

When attempting to rebalance sleep cycles, put yourself on a schedule that will become your drumbeat to live by. Aligning the body with a daily rhythm is as essential as learning to cope with stress and is often a missing link in insomnia treatment plans.

➢ Eat meals at a scheduled time.
➢ Go to bed around the same time as often as possible.
➢ Exercise regularly. Perhaps you used to be a swimmer or do yoga. Add them back in. If you feel incapable of that, walk

around the block or in your neighborhood. As simple as it sounds, it inspires great changes for many reasons. It connects people to their environment, and, if you do it year round, allows you to feel the seasons deeply.

For an even more coordinated plan, begin eating seasonally and take walks in all weather. I have found getting outside in all seasons, even if it's just for a few minutes in the depths of winter, makes for even more wondrous results.

Also, be aware that there are other elements in our lives that can contribute to insomnia and should be avoided 30-60 minutes before bed. They include: T.V., the computer, and foods that are high in simple sugars.

If you want something to do before hitting the sack, engage in activities that slow the mind down. Take a bath, write in a journal, take a slow walk around the block, knit, draw, or read. These don't work for everyone, but you could try a few or come up with your own.

And for those who can't seem to get tomorrow's tasks off their mind, this is also a good time to make a written list of those things and set it aside.

Chapter 10

Making and Using Your Portable and Natural First Aid Kit

Trauma occurs, and it shakes us. But with some basic ideas and tools, we can lessen the physical and emotional impact of traumatic situations.

This chapter will give ideas for putting together a first aid kit that can be used at home or condensed for hiking, backpacking, and travel. Also included are general strategies for dealing with some first aid situations. It's important to remember that plants can be valuable first aid tools on their own but are sometimes a prelude to seeking the help of a Western physician. In either case, herbs are an indispensible tool.

One of Our Family's First Aid Stories

In our household, it often feels that we are one step away from the emergency room. Accidents seem to occur in waves, from the Thank-Goodness-For-Bike-Helmets kind, to flying out of trees, broken bones or the simpler, but no less painful, sprains.

I recall one specific incident involving our youngest daughter, the counter, and a chopstick. At the impulsive age of four, she got out of her chair and approached the kitchen sink with a chopstick hanging out of her mouth. You are correct if your imagination allows you to picture what happened next. The chopstick lodged itself in the space between the counter and the lower cabinets. She impaled herself in the back of the throat.

To this day, I am amazed that we remained calm, for after I pulled the stick out, blood came gushing. We needed to stop it. The tricky part was the location. The back of the throat was no place to apply pressure. What I did was simple and worked beautifully.

Step 1: I gave her a glass of ice water. The cold decreased the pain and acted as a styptic and mild astringent. The bleeding decreased.

Step 2: As she drank the ice water, I made a quick strong infusion of yarrow, which took about five minutes. While I worked, I told her the story of how brave yarrow was and that it protected soldiers in battle and helped them heal their wounds. I mentioned that yarrow got its Latin name from Achilles, one of the best-known historical warriors.

She was transfixed. Stories about plants are fascinating and magical, especially to children. It's a great technique to use to keep kids calm. It works on adults, too.

By the time the story was over, the yarrow was ready to drink. She drank about 4 ounces of yarrow (I steeped 1 tablespoon of the dried herb in 4 ounces of hot water). The bleeding stopped within 20 seconds of drinking the tea, and the pain was greatly decreased. She ate dinner just fine.

That night before bed, I gave her more yarrow infusion with a bit of raspberry leaf and chamomile. I also added a few drops of St. John's wort and willow tincture as an anesthetic. I used this treatment plan for five days, giving her the infusion with tinctures two times daily.

My daughter was so excited to share her story with others. She didn't talk about being scared, the blood or pain. She talked about how brave she was, "just like Yarrow!"

Maladies the Kit Should Treat

An ideal first aid kit should prepare you for a variety of uses - a short hiking trip, a long backpacking trip, camping, a day at the park, or a drive across the country. Here is a list of needs to address:

1. Burns: chemical, heat, or sunburns
2. Topical injuries, such as splinters, bruises, puncture wounds with excessive bleeding, scrapes, lacerations, and topical infections (both fungal, bacteria, and abscesses)

3. Healing broken bones
4. Bug bites and stings
5. Muscle strain and sprains
6. The following acute situations: headaches, fever, acute respiratory infections, afflictions of the stomach and digestive tract (flu, food poisoning, gas and bloating, diarrhea, constipation)

Remedies to Pack

Choosing a handful of remedies and plants can be difficult. There are many excellent choices. So pick things that treat multiple ailments, lessening the load you carry. The following are items I like to have in my kit, and ones I highly recommend considering for your own. The list consists of two essential oils, two salves, a poultice, 3-4 tinctures, two homeopathic remedies, witch hazel, charcoal capsules, and a few other props.

Essential Oils

Lavender (*Lavendula angustifolia*) serves many purposes. Its properties are: analgesic, soothing nerve pain; anti-spasmodic for muscles topically; headaches, including migraines; insomnia and general relaxation; burns and sunburn; relieves itching and pain from bug bites and stings; and anti-bacterial.

For headaches, mix a drop of pure essential oil of lavender with a small amount of the Soothing Salve and apply to temples. Apply the same combination to the feet, wrists, and back of neck for relaxation or insomnia. To use lavender in the treatment of burns or sunburns, apply a few drops of pure essential oil undiluted (also known as neat) to the area to lessen inflammation, pain, and to speed healing. It may be applied neat to a sting or bug bite to aid pain and swelling as well. For eye irritation, put a drop of lavender in the palm of the hand and rub in. Cup your hand over your eye for a few minutes. Repeat throughout the day until the desired effect is achieved.

Tea tree (*Melaleuca alternifolia*) is known for its use in first aid kits. Its properties are: anti-septic; effective remedy for cold sores; infected wounds with puss and some fungal infections; effective gargle for respiratory and sinus infections, mouth infections, and to ease the pain of sore throats.

Tea tree can be applied neat to infections and cold sores. It can be used as a mouth rinse in a bit of water for mouth sores, sore throats, and respiratory and sinus infections. Gargle with a drop of tea tree in a bit of water three times daily. Inhalation is key for respiratory infections. Apply a drop to a hankie or something you are able to hold close to your face and breathe in. If you have access to a neti pot, add 1 drop of tea tree to your water. Do this one time daily until symptoms lessen.

Please Note: It is important to follow directions when using essential oils, especially if treating children, as they can be caustic to the skin and cause headaches when used excessively. A drop of essential oil goes a long way. Remember, there are many pounds of plant material accounted for in that little bottle.

The Salves

I carry two salves when I travel. One is the *Soothing Salve* for healing and soothing general scrapes, cuts, sunburn, and dry skin. It can also be used to dilute essential oils, thus eliminating the need to carry an extra bottle of carrier oil. The other is a salve that is strong and may be used for many things, from muscle strain to coughs to bug bites. It is the *Anti-inflammatory Salve.*

For instructions on how to make a salve, please refer back to Chapter 4. If you prefer to purchase salves or don't have the time to make them, I recommend a container of Tiger Balm to replace the Anti-inflammatory Salve, and a nice soothing calendula salve without comfrey to replace the Soothing Salve.

The Soothing Salve

Ingredients for the Soothing Salve are simple. The carrier oils I use are 1 part St. John's wort infused oil, 1 part calendula infused oil, and 1 part jojoba oil. The three essential oils I use in this salve are geranium, tea tree, and lavender. In 8 ounces of salve base, add 10 drops of each essential oil. That is about a 3/4% dilution.

This salve has many uses, is pleasantly scented, and is not irritating. It is appropriate for all ages. Apply it to scrapes, irritated skin, sunburns, mild fungal infections, and bruises. It can also be used in puncture wounds and deep gashes, as it will help keep infection at bay, and anesthetizes pain without healing too quickly. Reapply as needed for best results.

The Anti-inflammatory Salve

The Anti-inflammatory Salve serves a variety of specific purposes. It is made with quite a few essential oils and is strong and stimulating. This salve is made at 1.42% dilution of essential oils to salve (that's 80 total drops of pure essential oil to 8 ounces of salve base).

The carrier oils are 1 part St. John's wort infused oil, 1 part arnica infused oil, 1 part jojoba oil. The essential oils with the number of drops of each are: ginger (10), eucalyptus (25), rosemary (15), clove (10), oregano (10), geranium (10), and lavender (10).

The Anti-inflammatory Salve will treat many ailments such as arthritis and joint pain, muscle strain, sprains, bruises, bug bites and stings (aids itching, swelling and irritation), rubbed on the feet and chest in the event of a respiratory infection as a respiratory anti-spasmodic, headaches that are not heat-related, and topically for fungal infections.

Note: This salve is *not* intended for use on cuts, scrapes, rashes, punctures, or gaping wounds.

Poultice

A poultice is a heated, wet compress assembled in gauze that is applied to an affected area. It can consist of clay, ground herbs, essential oils, and herbal tinctures. It should be left on until cool, and then it must be reheated and reapplied until there is suitable change in the injury.

A poultice is used for drawing out pus, splinters and stingers that are sunken in too deep, and to reduce swelling. This one can also be used dry as a powder for damp feet with fungus, on irritated skin, or in a wound that is bleeding badly. It is anti-bacterial as well.

The poultice I carry with me in a little zip lock baggie contains the following: 2 parts cosmetic clay, to 1 part each of ground herbs of plantain leaf, marshmallow root, yarrow flowers, and myrrh resin. When I prepare the poultice for use, I add enough hot water to make a warm paste, add a dropper of echinacea tincture and a drop each of lavender and tea tree essential oil. Sandwich the warm, wet poultice between two pieces of gauze and apply. One can also lay over the poultice a piece of cloth soaked in hot water to maintain the heating element.

General Tinctures

Tinctures are an essential part of a first aid kit. How many I personally carry depends on the circumstances. Things I take into account are what my family generally needs, the season we are traveling in, and where we are going.

For general purposes, I tend to carry three different bottles with me. Here are some general ideas that one might consider. The size I take is either 1 or 2 ounces, and to pack them, I roll the glass tincture bottles up in a small cloth (which may come in handy for something else), and I pack them in zip lock baggies in case they break.

Bottle #1: Yarrow (*Achillea millefolium*) tincture, as a simple, is valuable in a first aid kit topically and internally. It is useful for diarrhea, heavy menstrual bleeding, and excessive bleeding internally and externally, to reduce fever, as an anti-inflammatory, to relieve headaches, for urinary tract infections, and sore throat.

Bottle #2: Ginger and Elderberry tincture (equal parts). This combination is powerful. Ginger (*Zingerber officinalis*) stimulates blood flow, is a warming and stimulating expectorant, anti-viral, improves digestion, anti-nausea, anti-inflammatory, and improves circulation. Elderberry (*Sambucus canadensis*) treats colds, flu, bronchial infections, is an anti-inflammatory anti-histamine due to the flavonoid, thereby reducing allergic symptoms and sinus irritation. Both plants stimulate immunity.

Bottle #3: Echinacea tincture (*Echinacea purpurea* or *angustifolia*) is a lymphatic herb that stimulates the body's innate ability to fight off acute illness by increasing white blood cell count and killer T-cells. Echinacea strengthens healthy cell integrity and increases macrophage count (immune cells located in the liver and lymphatic system) that help the body deal with waste produced by the body's fight against illness. It is a mild anti-bacterial internally and externally, and may be used internally and externally for snake bites or other poisonous insect bites, fevers, and for toothaches. For poisonous bites, apply to the bite, and take 30 drops every 15-30 minutes while getting to a doctor.

Other Ideas:

- Aller-tonic (a formula by Herbs Etc. for allergies, colds, or sinus infections)
- Blue vervain with feverfew (especially if you're prone to heat headaches with flushed red face)
- Yellow dock root (tones the bowel; low doses of about 5 drops stop diarrhea, while larger 15 drops doses help with constipation; improves digestion)
- Calendula with St. John's wort used topically to reduce pain from punctures or gaping wounds

For other tincture or plant ideas, please refer to the part of this chapter titled, *Applicable Strategies and Plants for First Aid.*

Homeopathic Remedies

There are two homeopathic remedies I use in my kit, especially if hiking. One is *Arnica montana*. It is a plant that is typically used externally to reduce swelling. Arnica stimulates circulation via the small capillaries, thus allowing the circulatory process to shuffle out the toxins causing the inflammation. When injuries occur, use the Anti-inflammatory Salve externally, and pellets of arnica homeopathic internally. Follow the dosage directions on the container.

The other homeopathic is poison ivy. If you are allergic to poison ivy and are exposed, take the homeopathic Rhus tox, 6 c.c. In some cases, it can very nearly stop the spreading and worsening of the condition. I recommend the Boiron brand. It can be found in most health and natural food stores. Follow the directions on the label for dosage.

Witch Hazel: Witch hazel extract (*Hamamelis virginiana*) has mild astringent, anti-septic, and anti-inflammatory properties. It is useful for diluting essential oils and is an excellent application for hemorrhoids, insect bites, and skin irritations. For relief from itching and poison ivy, add a few drops of lavender to witch hazel and apply liberally. Just remember, witch hazel is for topical application only, and should not be taken internally. Store it in a small plastic container.

Random Things to Add

Other helpful items to include in the kit are:

- Tea bags of raspberry leaf, peppermint, and chamomile (excellent quick plant poultices)
- Charcoal tablets (for food poisoning)
- Emergen-C (in the event there is major electrolyte loss from diarrhea, vomiting, or just hiking)
- Peppermint Altoids (helpful in a pinch for digestive woes and headaches)
- First aid items: band-aids in multiple sizes (including butterfly), tweezers, surgical tape, gauze, cotton, an eye rinse cup, and a small pair of scissors

Add a carry case of the appropriate size, and this portable natural first aid kit packs down very well. If you want to make it smaller, do. And remember, this is a basic kit that can be tailored to your own needs. Do you want to add something for constipation, parasites, or jet lag? Or perhaps you need less for hiking and more for city, like foot soaks from a long day walking on concrete or something more specific to your travel woes.

Warning: *This information is in no way to take the place of Western medical intervention. There are times when seeing a doctor is necessary. However, plants can help manage symptoms when you are on your way to the ER or doctor.*

Applicable Strategies and Plants for First Aid

- Abscesses
- Broken Bones
- Bruising and Sprains

- Deep injuries: cuts, gashes and puncture
- Digestive Distress - Quick Fixes

Plants in the *Materia medica* that will be helpful for other situations are plantain, garlic, and ginger.

Abscesses

Energetics needed: anesthetic, anti-bacterial, agents to open the wound, lymphatics, anti-septics, anti-inflammatory

Plants for internal use: usnea or goldenseal, echinacea or calendula, poke root

Plants for external use: tincture of blood root, yerba mansa (if you can get it), echinacea, myrrh, usnea, clove; essential oil or tincture in a base of sage, St. John's wort; arnica salve (may also use plain salve base with tinctures of St. John and arnica).

Note: Plantain works to open, but it is cooling and healing. I don't want to cool or heal. I want the abscess warm, open, and oozing.

Contraindicated: comfrey, calendula, and yarrow

Protocol

The smell of puss and infection is pretty intense, but you have to work past it. If the abscess is closed and hard, apply the salve gently about every 1-2 hours until the wound opens. Gently massage around the area to warm and loosen so the puss will release more easily.

Once open, gently massage around the wound to release it. Try not to inflict pain on the abscess sufferer. Once it has released a fair amount of puss, you will flush the wound. I use a clean dropper from an old tincture bottle. The dropper fits easily into the hole of the puncture or wound. The first flush should be salt water. Then I flush with that same tincture from above - myrrh, echinacea, clove, blood root, yerba mansa, and usnea. Use equal parts of everything except bloodroot, which I do at ½ part. Use the essential oils of myrrh and clove if you don't have their tinctures. You can also leave out the yerba mansa if needed but not the others.

Dilute 35 drops in 2 teaspoons of water, fill the dropper, insert it into the hole, and flushed out the wound. At the end of the treatment, I leave the fluid in the pocket for about half a minute while I massage around the wound. This does hurt a bit, especially on day one. But the herbs begin to numb and anesthetize the pain.

After this is done, give your suffer a lovely reward and apply the salve to the area with a few drops of the tincture formula mixed in.

Take tincture daily: usnea, poke root, calendula, echinacea - 35 drops 6 times a day for about 5 days. If improving, take it 3-4 times daily for about 5 more days.

Note: There are times when antibiotics are needed. In the case of Peritonsillar abscess or high fevers with abscess. That need should not be ignored. Do the gut and body rebuilding after. The bacteria in an abscess is anaerobic. They thrive in oxygen-deprived environments and replicate at a high rate of speed. If you don't have a fever, the wound is staying open and draining, and you have no reason to believe there is staph or MRSA, than you're probably good with the natural stuff. If, however, you are on immune suppressing drugs, have diabetes, or are elderly, have had or recently been exposed to MRSA, staph or strep, and/or have a depleted immune system, see a doctor please.

Broken Bones

Internal treatment for broken bones is straightforward. And remember, formulate based on need, or simply pick one plant to use. For external treatment, I refer you to the section on Bruising, Sprains, and Broken Bones below.

Internal for Bone Healing:

Comfrey leaf tea or homeopathic: Comfrey aids bone knitting. Follow dosing instructions on the homeopathic package. If drinking the tea (leaf only, NEVER the root), steep 1 teaspoon in 8 ounces of hot water for 5 minutes. You may also do the long cold infusion described in Chapter 3. Drink 4 ounces of the infusion 2 times a day. Only do the tea for 2 weeks.

Boneset tincture: Helps the bone set, literally, using the bone's ability to magnetically find the other piece. Take 3 drops 3 times a day for 4-6 weeks.

Solomon's seal and mullein flower tincture: These plants help relieve muscular and joint swelling that prevents the bone from setting. They are cooling and balancing to muscle tone, which helps to hold bone structure in place. Mullein flower is also a nervine.

Blue vervain: To help with blood re-absorption, balance circulation, and decrease constriction that can interfere with circulation and nervous system stress. Take 5-10 drops 3 times daily.

Bruising, Sprains, and Broken Bones

Severe bruising, sprains, and broken bones are painful. We use herbs both internally and externally to relieve pain, inflammation, and inspire the blood to re-absorb back into the circulatory system. If using plant remedies to support a bone break, use them in conjunction with medical treatment.

External Application:

Avoid touching or rubbing the area affected for as long as there is extreme swelling or pain. This depends on the severity of the injury. With breaks, you will not touch the break location. You can still apply topical remedies during this time, though. Put the formula around the circumference of area in distress, getting as close as possible. This will relieve inflammation, aid blood re-absorption, and help with pain. Apply 3-4 times daily. After two days, the area will probably be less painful, and you can gently apply herbal medicines directly to the area. Keep covered if needed.

Use:

Arnica and comfrey salve: Use a salve with the infused oils and supporting essential oils, like the Anti-inflammatory Salve mentioned in this chapter. There is an arnica homeopathic gel, but I prefer the salve with infused oil because anyone can make it!

Applying hot and cold is essential. Our doctor taught us to soak the area in a bucket of cold water from the tap as long as can be tolerated, alternately applying warmth. There is another way that I have successfully used hot and cold, but first, let's look at how the two function together, and why using one over the other is not usually a good idea with sprains and some breaks.

Most people haven't heard this, but studies show that using cold is controversial in injuries, because cold disables the immune system, and our body's ability to repair damage. With sprains and breaks, however, cold helps excessive heat and inflammation. Excessive is the key word here. If inflammation and heat are too extreme, it also disables immunity. Cold in the instance of severe sprains and some breaks helps maintain heat to functional levels, so our immune system, and circulatory system can repair damage, promote healing, relieve swelling, and assists the removal of cell die off (something that can exacerbate the condition at hand).

I have come up with other methods that employ hot and cold. In some cases, I have applied a warming salve before submerging the area affected in a cold bath. And when it comes to tricky to treat areas, like broken collar bones, I have used a warming and cooling salve alternately to relieve inflammation. The warming salve is the same one quoted above. The cooling salve uses peppermint and lavender pure essential oils. The infused oils that make up this salves base are specific for broken bones. They are infused oils of mullein leaf and flower, and Solomon's seal oil. These plants help relieve muscular swelling that prevents the bone from setting. As mentioned above, these plants are cooling and balancing to muscle tone, which helps hold bone structure in place.

Always apply a warming salve after a cold bath of the area. Keep the area covered to help maintain warmth.

Poultices (not for broken bones or first few days of severe bruising): Plant poultices can be useful. They can be applied warm or at room temperature. I use tea bags full of herbs for small bruises and muslin cloth laid with soaked herbs for larger areas. Plants to include are blue vervain, comfrey leaf, yarrow, and calendula. Again, to maintain heat, place a wet cloth as warm as can be tolerated or a heating pad on its lowest setting, if tolerated.

Internal Remedies:

Blue vervain and yarrow tincture: To help with blood re-absorption, balance blood circulation, and decrease constriction that can interfere with circulation and nervous system stress. Take 5 drops of each 3 times daily.

Arnica homeopathic: To increase small capillary circulation, thereby decreasing inflammation and swelling by improving blood flow. Follow the dosage instructions on the label.

Deep Injuries: cuts, gashes, and punctures

Energetics needed: anti-inflammatory, hemostatic/styptic, anti-bacterial and anti-microbial, anesthetic, cell regenerative

Plants for internal use: lymphatics (echinacea or calendula), anti-bacterial if needed (usnea, goldenseal), arnica homeopathic

Plants for external use: Salves of calendula and St. John's wort with lavender and tea tree essential oil; a soak or basting of yarrow tea with a few of the following: echinacea, calendula, St. John's wort, usnea or goldenseal tinctures (per ½ cup of tea, about 15 drops of each tincture); can also add lavender essential oil (about 3 drops in that ½ cup of yarrow tea), arnica tincture (a few drops in the yarrow tea, see below)

Contraindicated: comfrey

Protocol

The cut, puncture, or gash occurs - apply pressure if you can, and run cold water over the area. I often put a drop of lavender in this process if I can, but there is not always time, space or the opportunity.

Have someone make the yarrow for you. If you can't, use the tincture of yarrow. About 60 drops of tinctures in 4 ounces of cool water is good.

To make the infusion: 3 tablespoons of yarrow in 4 ounces of hot water; steep for 10 minutes if you can.

While it steeps, put 35 drops each of St. John's wort tincture and calendula tincture in 2 tablespoons of cold water. Put it on! Sometimes basting the wound is great. Use a syringe or turkey baster. Wash the cut with the solution using a syringe, dousing the herbs over the wound repeatedly for about a minute. The pain will begin to dissipate. In these situations, depending on severity, complete pain relief can be felt in 3-30 minutes (with very deep gashes 30 minutes).

St. John's wort and calendula anesthetize nerve pain quickly. I have used them on deep puncture wounds for the same reason. Calendula tincture is also anti-bacterial, demulcent, and a lymphatic stimulant.

Icing the strained yarrow solution, baste the wound. Yarrow stops it after about 20 seconds. If swelling is bad, add a couple drops of arnica tincture to the solution.

If you remember the story of my daughter puncturing the back of her throat with a chopstick, you remember yarrow. It's anti-inflammatory, hemostatic (stops bleeding) and helps with pain in tissue.

If stitches are needed, by all means get them. I have gotten them and not gotten them. Also, keep in mind that if you sever nerves, it can take 1-1 ½ years for nerves to regenerate. You may feel prickly sensations as the feeling comes back to an area. That is normal.

I have seen untreated gashes abscess. If that occurs, the wound has to be opened up. Refer to the abscess section. And please seek medical attention if there are fevers or streaks coming from the injury.

Healing: Watch the wound daily for infection. Epsom salt soaks can be helpful. Healing salves that are used should be simple: calendula, St. John's infused oil with lavender and tea tree essential oil. (Remember - no comfrey leaf or root!)

Digestive Distress – Quick Fixes

Digestive distress comes in many forms when traveling and can greatly affect the quality of one's trip. Food and water borne illnesses, constipation, diarrhea, gas, spasms, and bloating are the most common complaints. The cause is often due to the fact that people eat differently when they travel. And whether that means eating poorly or having a food adventure, the results can be the same.

Here are some symptom and malady specific remedies. Formulate for your specific needs.

Food and water borne illnesses: Take 5 drops of goldenseal tincture, 5 drops of black walnut hull tincture, and swallow 1 small clove of garlic sliced 3 times daily until symptoms improve. See the other symptoms for further support.

Food poisoning: **tincture of** blue vervain, peppermint, and goldenseal; take about 5-10 drops 3-4 times daily

Constipation: tincture of culvers root, dandelion root, and ginger root, or yellow dock root tincture; take 5-10 drops 3-4 times daily

Diarrhea: I often recommend diarrhea be allowed to run its course to a certain degree. If one is in danger of dehydration or needs to control the symptom due to travel or sleep, try some of these remedies.

- 3 cups daily of raspberry leaf tea or 10-20 drops of the tincture 3-4 times daily; 5 drops of yellow dock root tincture

- 20 drops of yarrow tincture with 10 drops of raspberry leaf tincture
- 5 drops each of yellow dock root and red root tincture 3-4 times daily
- Use herbal teas with honey or Emergen-C to prevent dehydration.

Acid reflux: 5 drops each of chamomile, licorice root, and catnip tincture, taken 4 times daily between meals

Poor digestion from poor quality food (without acid reflux): 5 drops each of culvers root, dandelion root, and ginger root tincture, taken 3-4 times daily with meals

Anti-spasmodics: catnip tincture, ginger tea, peppermint tea - drink 2-3 cups daily before meals or at the onset of symptoms; take 10-35 drops of catnip and motherwort tincture up to 4 times in 1-2 hours until symptoms subside. A maintenance dose is 10-15 drops 3-4 times daily.

Carminatives for gas and bloating: ginger tea, fennel seeds chewed, as a tea or a tincture

Section 3

Materia medica: Chapters 11-13

Chapter 11

Internal Plant Medicines *Materia medica*

Information on each plant is organized in the following format:

Common name (*Latin name*) - **Taste**, **Energetics**, **Organ System Affinity.**

> **Contraindications**
> **Part of plant used**
> **Plant family**
> **Used fresh, dried, or both**
> **Best menstruums for extraction**
> **Medicine making dilutions**
> **Dosage**

Here I may include basic information on namesake or history.

- ➢ Uses
- • Sample Formulas

It's important to remember that the formulas and dosages given with each plant are examples. You may see different ideas in other books, and you may have ideas of your own.

Anise hyssop (*Agastache spp.*) - **Taste**: sweet, pungent-minty, licorice, aromatic. **Energetics**: analgesic to head, heart, and chest from excessive coughing, diaphoretic, anti-microbial, expectorant, carminative. **Organ System Affinity:** stomach, head, immune, respiratory tract.

> **Contraindications:** none known
> **Part of plant used**: flower and leaves (no stems)
> **Plant family:** Lamiaceae (mint family)
> **Used fresh, dried, or both**: both
> **Best menstruums for extraction:** alcohol, honey, water
> **Medicine making dilutions:** fresh plant tincture, 1:2; dried plant tincture, 1:5 (60% alcohol, 40% water); tea - 1-2 teaspoons per cup

Dosage: acute tincture dosage, 5-10 drops 3-4 times daily; acute tea dosage, 2-3 cups daily; tonic tincture dosage, 3-5 drops 3-4 times daily

Anise hyssop is native to North America and was widely used by many native tribes. It is a relative to hyssop (*Hyssopus officinalis*), but both are quite different in nature. Hyssop means 'holy herb.'

Uses:

> Colds and flus, as a tea or tincture; relieves fever and stomach pains, as a mild expectorant
> Relieves pain in head, chest, and heart from excessive coughing
> For low to high fevers
> Food poisoning
> Used to flavor other less appealing medicines

Sample Formulas:

- Cold and flu: tea with yarrow and elderflower
- Tincture: with yarrow, and elecampane
- Food poisoning: tea with peppermint; tincture with peppermint and blue vervain
- Bronchitis or other painful chest infection: tincture with lobelia, Solomon's seal, elecampane

Basil (*Ocimum basilicum*) - **Taste:** sweet, pungent, aromatic, warming. **Energetics:** diaphoretic, anti-viral, expectorant, circulatory stimulant, cerebral stimulant, anti-oxidant, anti-inflammatory, carminative, anti-viral, galactagogue, emmenagogue, adaptogen. **Organ System Affinity**: immune, stomach, nervous system, adrenals, mind/head, lungs, skin, circulatory system, women's reproductive system.

Contraindications: none known
Part of plant used: flowers, leaves, and non-woody stems
Plant family: Lamiaceae (mint family)
Used fresh, dried, or both: fresh for tincturing; dried for tea
Best menstruums for extraction: alcohol, oil, water, or honey
Medicine making dilutions: fresh tincture, 1:2; for tea, add 1-2 teaspoons to 8 ounces of water and steep covered for 15

minutes. Note: Basil is an aromatic plant. Its volatile/aromatic oils will evaporate easily. Steep covered, and do not boil the leaves.

Dosage: acute tincture dosage, 5-15 drops 3-4 times daily; acute tea dosage, 2-3 cups daily; tonic tincture dosage, 5-10 drops 3-4 times daily

The species name for basil, *basilicum*, has two interpretations, each one identifying basil's dual reputations historically. For in some old cultures, basil is revered and honored, while in others it is feared and considered evil.

According to Nicolas Culpeper, *basilicum* is derived from the Greek word *basilicon*, calling to attention the relationship of basil to a basilisk, an enormous snake like creature with a venomous bite and the ability to kill with a look. Maude Grieve says that the term *basilicum* was derived from the Greek word for king, *basileus*. She says that it was thought that "the scent was fit for a king" and that it was used in unguents made for royalty.

Uses:

> A use from Culpepper – to draw venom from poisonous bites ("Every like draws his like")
> Upper respiratory infections, helps reduce fever, warm the blood, stimulate circulation, is an anti-viral and mild expectorant
> For poor digestion, helps dispel gas and bloating; helps expectorate mucus from the colon
> As a tea, an anti-oxidant anti-inflammatory that assists cell repair and protects cells, therefore improving function
> Circulatory and cerebral stimulant, relieving cloudy headedness, and lifting mood
> Helps instill proper sleep cycles and mood balance during the day as it balances the secretion of cortisol
> Helps stimulate mild production for nursing
> Will assist the after birth being expelled and acts as an emmenagogue
> Excellent in anti-inflammatory rubs for external use infused oil

Sample Formulas:

- Cold or flu: tea of basil, yarrow, ginger; tincture of basil, yarrow, elecampane
- Drawing venom: fresh leaves of plantain and basil, chewed and applied
- Poor digestion: tea of basil, cardamom seeds and catnip; tincture of basil, catnip, yellow dock root
- Mental clarity: tea of basil, rosemary, peppermint; tincture of basil, rosemary, peppermint
- Anti-oxidant tea: long infusion of basil, rosehips, cilantro

Blue vervain (*Verbena hastata or stricta*) - **Taste**: acrid bitter. **Energetics**: sedative, relaxing diaphoretic, diuretic, bitter tonic, mild anti-spasmodic, anti-anxiety, anti-inflammatory for headaches, aphrodisiac. **Organ System Affinity**: spine and nervous system, urinary tract, stomach, immune system, head, adrenals.

Contraindications: dry eczema and psoriasis (from client experience); sometimes high blood pressure medications
Part of plant used: leaves and flowering tops (stems removed)
Plant family: Verbenaceae
Used fresh, dried, or both: I believe blue vervain and hoary vervain are best used/made as a fresh plant tincture. If you use it dried, be sure it is less than a year old and was stored properly. I also find the tincture is more effective than the tea.
Best menstruums for extraction: alcohol (it is so bitter, the tea is difficult to consume for most)
Medicine making dilutions: Fresh plant tincture, 1:2 (add no water); dried plant tincture, 1:5 (70% alcohol, 30% distilled water)
Tincture dosage: for ages five and up as a tonic for chronic conditions, 3-15 drops 2-4 times daily (lower doses for lower ages); for acute conditions, 5-20 drops for ages five and up 3-4 times daily

According to Maude Grieve, vervain is derived from the Celtic *ferfaen- fer*, 'to drive away,' and *faen*, 'a stone,' a name that identifies its ability to expel urinary gravel. The Iroquois tribe used the plant to drive away individuals who were obnoxious, also reflective of the 'to drive away' purpose of the plant, though they had no knowledge of the Celtic meaning. *Verbena* translates as 'altar plant,' a title possibly given by Roman priests who believed it was one plant responsible for healing the wounds of Christ on the Mount of Calvary.

Uses:

> High fevers associated with acute illness and low-grade fevers that are chronic and associated with autoimmune disease
> Food poisoning
> Headaches associated with flu, high fever, PMS, high hot headaches that radiate from tightness in the spine and/or neck
> Blue vervain is an acrid bitter, sometimes making one shiver as it relaxes the nervous system. I have seen strong men quake after taking just a few simple drops. I use it for nervous system agitation that results in exhaustion, periods of depression and anxiety, and tension in the upper body.
> Nervine for autoimmune conditions: chronic fatigue, fibromyalgia, multiple sclerosis, Chron's
> Unbreakable patterns of tightness in nervous system/spine – recycles energy from nerves to adrenals
> Iroquois use it for heat sickness in summer
> Kidney stones
> Blue vervain relaxes nerves that are functioning in excess, allows energy to disperse, increasing blood circulation (not by heating and stimulating, though), opens the pores of the skin, and supports digestive and urinary function.

Sample Formulas:

- Kidney stones: tincture of blue vervain, gravel root, cleavers, hydrangea root, yarrow, or shepherds purse (for bleeding)
- High fever: tincture of blue vervain, yarrow, catnip
- High hot headaches: tincture of feverfew and blue vervain
- Autoimmune nervine formula: blue vervain, skullcap
- Food poisoning: blue vervain, anise hyssop, peppermint

Calendula (*Calendula officinalis*) - **Taste**: sweet, acrid bitter, pungent, salty, warm and stimulating to lymph, relaxing to nerves, moistening but toning to tissue. **Energetics**: diaphoretic, styptic, anti-septic, anti-fungal, anti-bacterial, astringent, lymphatic, anti-oxidant, nervine, anti-inflammatory, emollient and demulcent, anesthetic. **Organ System Affinity**: liver, eyes, lymph, nerves, skin, immune system, blood.

> **Contraindications**: should not be used for chronic conditions when the person is prone to edema
> **Part of plant used**: flowering tops (can use stems, too, but it will re-flower if you only pinch the flowers)
> **Plant family:** Asteraceae (composite family)
> **Used fresh, dried, or both:** both
> **Best menstruums for extraction:** alcohol and oil (if using water, it will lack resins and anti-bacterial agents)
> **Medicine making dilutions**: fresh plant tincture or oil, 1:2 (add no water); dried plant tincture, 1:5 (70% alcohol, 30% distilled water)
> **Tincture dosage:** for ages 1 and up as a tonic for chronic conditions, 2-10 drops 2-4 times daily (lower doses for lower ages); for acute conditions, 5-15 drops 2-4 times daily
> **Tea dosage**: 2 teaspoons of dried flower steeped in 8 ounces of water for 10 minutes

Calendula officinalis has been in use as a medicine for thousands of years. The name Calendula is derived from the Latin *calendea,* meaning 'calendar,' a name that reflects the unique trait of this plant to flower throughout the year.

Uses:

> ➢ This plant is specific for use on acute bacterial and viral infections. It stimulates the immune system, is anti-inflammatory to irritated tissue, anesthetizes pain, is diaphoretic, and decreases glandular swelling.
> ➢ As a tonic for recurrent tonsillitis and/or strep throat
> ➢ Topical: bug bites, rashes-diaper and general irritation, vaginitis, in lymphatic formula for swellings (see Chapter 12, Infused Oil *Materia medica* for more details)
> ➢ Jaundice with swollen liver
> ➢ As a pungent and resinous plant, calendula can penetrate lymphatic swellings that are hard. It is specific for this hardness especially when decreased immunity and recurrent acute infections are a problem. It can assist the softening of the hardness, and it increases lymphatic circulation. The balance it brings to tissue and fluid transport creates a terrain that does not support illness, thereby acting as a tonic.

> Nerve pain and damage internally and externally; it is used interchangeably with St. John's wort (see Chapter 12, Infused Oil *Materia medica* for more details)

Sample Formulas:

- Recurrent tonsillitis or strep throat: tincture of calendula, echinacea, and poke root
- Jaundice with swollen liver: tincture of calendula, yellow dock root, and milk thistle
- Lymphatic swelling with recurrent infections: tincture of calendula, echinacea, poke root
- Acute bacterial infection (strep): tincture of calendula, cleavers, echinacea, usnea, poke root or stillingia
- Acute viral infection (tonsillitis): tincture of calendula, cleavers, echinacea, poke root or stillingia

Catnip (*Nepeta cataria*) - **Taste:** Pungent, aromatic, acrid bitter, relaxant, and warming to cool. **Energetics:** carminative, anti-spasmodic, relaxing diaphoretic, sedative, nervine tonic; contains a small amount of resins that, in tincture form, allow the plant act as a very mild demulcent, anti-inflammatory for headaches. **Organ System Affinity:** nervous system, digestive system, uterus, and respiratory tract.

Contraindications: none known
Part of plant used: flowers and leaves (no stems)
Plant family: Lamiaceae (mint family)
Used fresh, dried, or both: fresh is best; dried if less than 8 months old
Best menstruums for extraction: alcohol or water
Medicine making dilutions: fresh tincture, 1:2; dried tincture, 1:5 (60% alcohol, 40% alcohol); tea, 1-2 teaspoons steeped in 8 ounces of water covered for 10 minutes
Dosage: tincture, 2-10 drops 3-4 times daily; tea, 1-2 teaspoons steeped in 8 ounces of hot water covered for 10 minutes drunk 2-3 times daily

According to the book titled *The Names of Plants* by D. Gledhill, the name, *Nepeta cataria*, is derived from place and animal. Nepi, Italy was an ancient city where catnip grew in great abundance. *Nepeta* is in reference to that city and was a name Pliny, the great Roman naturalist and writer who lived from 23-79 AD, first coined. *Cataria* is Latin for 'of cats.'

Uses:

> ➤ Specific indications for use in the digestive tract: Irritable Bowel Syndrome with anxiety and nervousness, anti-spasmodic for colic, helps relieve gas and bloating. It is my experience that people who are very tense and anxious can hold their emotions in their stomach. This causes wind/gas and tension/constriction. Catnip is carminative, therefore relieves wind, while relaxing muscles and nerves. For a secondary effect, its bitter properties can mildly stimulate gastric secretions and the liver, thereby improving digestion.
> ➤ Insomnia with or without gastrointestinal issues
> ➤ Relaxing diaphoretic for low and high fevers, especially helpful when the child or adult cannot break a sweat
> ➤ Anti-spasmodic in lungs, useful for bronchitis when a sleep aid is needed

Sample Formulas:

- Colic in infants and children: tincture or tea of catnip and fennel
- Gastrointestinal distress with jaundice: fennel, catnip, yellow dock root
- Gastrointestinal distress with excess hydrochloric acid secretions: catnip and chamomile
- Mild insomnia: tincture of catnip, passionflower, skullcap
- High fever formula with an inability to sweat: tea or tincture of catnip, linden, yarrow with tincture of blue vervain (if fever won't manage)
- Bronchitis: tincture of catnip, lobelia, elecampane, Solomon's seal with marshmallow root tea (if the cough is dry), and osha root tincture (if the cough is too wet)
- Colds that sit in the lungs: tea of ginger, catnip, thyme
- Headaches that are high and hot: tincture of catnip, blue vervain, and (if migraine like) feverfew

Camomille (*Anthemis nobilis*) - **Taste**: aromatic bitter, pungent, sweet. **Energetics**: demulcent and emollient, carminative, nervine, potent anti-inflammatory, anti-spasmodic, sedative, diuretic, mucosal tonic (speeds healing of skin and mucous membranes of the stomach and colon), antacid, ulcer protective, mild anti-bacterial, mild anti-fungal, mild relaxing diaphoretic, inactivates toxins produced by bacterial die off, emmenagogue. **Organ System Affinity**: stomach, skin, urinary tract, nervous system, mucous membranes, uterus.

Contraindications: underproduction of hydrochloric acid
Part of plant used: flowers
Plant family: Asteraceae (composite family)
Used fresh, dried, or both: both
Best menstruums for extraction: alcohol, oil, water, or honey
Medicine making dilutions: fresh tincture, 1:2; dried tincture, 1:5 (60% alcohol, 40% water); tea, 1 tablespoon steeped for 10 minutes in 8 ounces hot water
Dosage: tincture, 5-10 drops 2-4 times daily; Tea, 2-3 cups daily

In the Middle Ages, chamomile, also known as maythen, was considered one of *The Nine Sacred Herbs*. The others are mugwort, waybroad (plantain), stime (watercress), atterlothe *(Eschiem vulgare)*, wergulu (nettle), crabapple, chervil, and fennel.

According to Maude Grieve, chamomile was once called 'ground apple' due to its apple like scent. The name was derived from the Greek words *kamai*, meaning 'on the ground,' and *melon*, 'an apple.'

Uses:

- ➢ Used as a sleep aid for the ill and infirmed by monks of the Middle Ages, who would line the beds of sick folk to inspire good rest and restore wellness
- ➢ When hydrochloric is in excess, this is an excellent plant ally. It is also a carminative to aid gas and bloating, anti-spasmodic, relieves heart burn, protects and speeds healing of the mucous membranes in the stomach and colon, is ulcer protective, demulcent to sooth irritation, reduces inflammation, inactivates toxins from bacterial die off, and is ant-spasmodic.

➢ As the tea and tincture are mildly bitter, it has a slightly stimulating effect on the liver.
➢ Excellent for anxiety with high blood pressure and stomach distress that is stress induced
➢ Aids restoration of healthy bowel flora and increases the colon's ability to heal from *Candida* overgrowth when taken with acidophilus by reducing inflammation and speeding healing
➢ Nervine tonic - excellent for insomnia with high blood pressure and gastrointestinal issues
➢ Colic in infants with acid reflux
➢ Teething pain with emotional and gastrointestinal distress in infants
➢ Hysteria in children
➢ The tea or oil makes an excellent skin wash or application for dryness, red patchy inflammation and irritation; is emollient, anti-inflammatory and speeds healing
➢ As a tea for nervousness with PMS and the inability of the period to be stimulated; helps promote menstrual flow and reduce uterine pain
➢ Chamomile is a relaxant. Much like blue vervain, in relaxing the nervous system, it has a stimulating effect on the circulation of blood.

Sample Formulas:

• Soak for skin: tea of chamomile and marshmallow root
• Excess hydrochloric acid: tea of chamomile and fennel, sipped slowly 3-4 times daily between meals
• Chronic *Candida*: tincture of chamomile, black walnut hull, yellow dock root, calendula
• Infant colic: glycerin tincture of chamomile (only if acid reflux is present), catnip, fennel

Cleavers (*Galium aparine*) - **Taste**: salty, sweet, cool, and moistening; relaxes the nerves, but stimulates lymphatic circulation. **Energetics**: diuretic, anti-inflammatory in the lymphatic system and urinary tract, alterative, nervine tonic. **Organ System Affinity:** urinary tract, nervous system, immune system, blood, lymphatic system.

Contraindications: none known
Part of plant used: stems, leaves ,and flowering tops (top 8 inches)
Plant family: Rubiaceae (flowering plant or coffee family)
Used fresh, dried, or both: As a lymphatic, it must be used fresh; as a nervine, it can be drunk dried as a tea.
Best menstruums for extraction: alcohol, or juicing it, pouring it into an ice cube tray and freezing it, water (for nervine effect)
Medicine making dilutions: fresh tincture, 1:2; dried tea, 1 ounce of herb in 8 ounces of hot water steeped for 10 minutes
Dosage: 5-15 drops 3-4 times daily

Gallium aparine is known by many common names, as most herbs are. The problem is that many of them are still used. You will find it listed as *clivers* in Maude Grieve's book, hear it referred to as *bedstraw* by those who have observed deer using it for a mattress, and *sticky weed* by farmers who find it annoying. *Aparine* is of the Greek word *aparo*, meaning 'to seize,' referring to the sticky nature of the plant and its ability to simply reach out and grab your leg. Not to worry, it doesn't hurt.

Uses:

> ➢ Non irritating diuretic for urinary tract infection
> ➢ Formulas for recurrent strep
> ➢ Chronic skin conditions that are hot, red, and raised (psoriasis, eczema, scabies)
> ➢ Reduces lymphatic swellings, both hard and soft
> ➢ Specific for cancer treatment and post therapy to improve the lymph duct's ability to filter and clean the lymph fluid
> ➢ In cases of Irritable Bowel Syndrome and Disease when there are bright red skin rashes and chronic food allergies/intolerances
> ➢ According to Maude Grieve, the seeds were once used as a coffee substitute. This reflects its relationship to the coffee tree, but also reflects the stimulating nature of the plant on the lymphatic system.

Sample Formulas:

> • Urinary tract infection: tincture of cleavers, yarrow (if bleeding), pipsissewa
> • Nervine tea: dried cleavers with oat straw

- Chronic skin inflammations: tincture of cleavers, burdock seed, nettle seed
- Strep throat: tincture of usnea, cleavers, calendula, echinacea, poke root
- General post cancer treatment: tinctures of cleavers, red root, plantain; tea of cleavers, plantain, raspberry leaf
- General lymphatic and blood tonic: tincture of cleavers, violet leaf, red root

Echinacea (*Echinacea purpurea* or *angustifolia*) - **Taste**: sweet, warm, and stimulating. **Energetics**: astringent, anti-microbial, immune modulator, anti-inflammatory, anti-diarrheal, anti-viral, analgesic. **Organ System Affinity**: lymphatic and immune system, joints, nerves, blood.

Contraindications: autoimmune disease (due to immune stimulating effects); immune suppressing drugs
Part of plant used: seeds, flower, stem, leaves, root
Plant family: Asteraceae (aster /sunflower/composite family)
Used fresh, dried, or both: both
Best menstruums for extraction: alcohol for immune boosting, water for polysaccharides
Medicine making dilutions: fresh tincture, 1:2; dried tincture, 1:5 (50% alcohol, 50% water); tea, 1-3 teaspoons steeped for 15 minutes
Dosage: tincture for acute infection, 5-20 drops 3-4 times daily; tea for acute infection, 2-3 cups daily; tincture for tonic long term use, 3-5 drops 4 times daily

According Dr. Kelly Kindscher, it was an 18th century German botanist by the name of Conrad Moenoch who named the echinacea plant. The term is derived from the Greek *echinos*, meaning 'hedgehog,' and deemed so for its rounded spiny seed head. Latin species name *angustifolia* is from two Latin terms - *angust*, meaning 'narrow' and *foli*, which translates as 'leaf.' *Purpurea* refers to the plant's purple ray of flowers.

Uses:

➤ Echinacea is a lymphatic herb that stimulates the body's innate ability to fight off acute illness by increasing white blood cell count and killer T-cells. It strengthens healthy cell

integrity and increases macrophage count (immune cells located in the liver and lymphatic system) that help the body deal with waste produced by the body's fight against illness.
- ➤ Swellings: joints, lymphatic ducts, hemorrhoids, abscesses, boils
- ➤ Septicemia with antibiotics
- ➤ Apply locally for toothache
- ➤ As a tonic to the person who suffers from chronic acute infections of the respiratory tract (upper and lower), both bacterial and viral. These infections are a sign that the blood is phlegm, thick, and too cold, and that immunity is low.
- ➤ Bronchitis, pneumonia, strep infections, ear infections, and sinusitis, especially when mucous is thick and stuck, or the immune system is having trouble rallying to fight the infection
- ➤ Infections of the gastrointestinal tract, diarrhea, shigellosis
- ➤ In formulas for rheumatism
- ➤ As an internal tonic and external application for bites from venomous bugs, spiders, and snakes

Sample Formulas:

- Bronchitis: tincture of echinacea, elecampane, Solomon's seal, lobelia
- Strep throat: echinacea, calendula, cleavers, usnea, poke root
- Shigellosis: tincture of echinacea, goldenseal, anise hyssop
- Rheumatism: tincture of echinacea, turmeric, black cohosh; tea of echinacea and oat straw
- Ear infections: tincture of echinacea, St. John's wort, cayenne, usnea (if bacterial), elecampane (if sinuses are involved)

Elderberry (*Sambucus canadensis*) - **Taste**: sour, sweet, pungent, stimulating, warming. **Energetics:** diaphoretic, diuretic, anti-viral, expectorant, anti-spasmodic, anti-oxidant (high in flavonoids), anti-inflammatory, cathartic, aperients (laxative). **Organ System Affinity:** immune system, lungs, sinuses, joints, urinary tract, circulatory system.

Contraindications: autoimmune disease, as it is an immune modulator (stimulates the immune system); high fevers (according to Michael Moore)

Part of plant used: the black berries (not red, for they are toxic to humans), flowers (mainly diaphoretic and milder), leaves (externally); detach stems, as the stems, twigs, bark and root are high in cyanide.
Quote from Michael Moore: *"Flower, berries and leaf, will never bring you grief;*
Bark and root for teas, will bring you to your knees."
Plant family: Caprifoliaceae (honeysuckle family)
Used fresh, dried, or both: both
Best menstruums for extraction: alcohol, oil, honey, and water
Medicine making dilutions: fresh or dried in alcohol or honey – fresh, 1:2; dried, 1:5 (60% alcohol, 50% water)
Dosage: Acute illness, 5-20 drops of tincture 3-6 times daily or 1 teaspoon steeped for 20 minutes in 8 ounces hot water drunk 2-3 times daily

Maude Grieve tells us that *Sambucus* is derived from the Greek term *sambuca*, which was used by the writer Pliny (243-79 A.D.) and other ancients to refer to the Sackbut. It was thought that the wood of the elder was used in its construction. Elder comes from the Anglo-Saxon word *aeld*, which means 'fire.'

Uses:

> ➤ Cherokee medicine: rheumatism - salve for boils and burns (not sure which part was used, but I assume flowers), leaves for a wash for sores
> ➤ Cold and flu with low-grade fevers, nasal and lung mucous that is thick and stuck
> ➤ Colds with a cough that just won't quit
> ➤ Anti-oxidant for cell repair with fragile capillaries
> ➤ Sore throats
> ➤ Flowers: an excellent diaphoretic, and excellent medicine for sore eyes

Sample Formulas:

- Cold and flu (without high fever): tincture of elderberry, echinacea, osha; tea of ginger, elderberry, yarrow, echinacea
- Cold with cough: tincture of elderberry, peppermint, elecampane, elderberry, peppermint, ginger
- Capillary repair: tea of elderberry, rose hips, raspberry leaf

- Bronchitis with low-grade fever and dry stuck mucous: tincture of elderberry, elecampane, Solomon's seal

Elecampane (*Inula helenium*) - **Taste**: pungent, aromatic bitter, warming and balancing to tissue tone. **Energetics**: diaphoretic, expectorant, decongestant, anti-spasmodic, cholagogue, emmenagogue, diuretic, anti-parasitic. **Organ System Affinity**: liver, colon, lungs, sinuses, kidney, and bladder.

> **Contraindications**: pregnancy
> **Part of plant used**: root
> **Plant family**: Asteraceae (sunflower family)
> **Used fresh, dried, or both**: both
> **Best menstruums for extraction**: alcohol
> **Medicine making dilutions**: fresh tincture, 1:2, dried tincture, 1:5 (70% alcohol, 30% water)
> **Dosage**: tonic long term, 5-10 drops 3-4 times daily; acute illness, 15-35 drops 3-5 times daily

Elecampane is a tall plant, growing 4-5 feet in height. The leaves are quite large, too. They are about four inches across and a foot long. The flower is resinous and golden, while the root of this plant appears to have oil ducts and looks and feels a bit like skin. I feel this is a clear indication that it is useful for toning tissue. While many historical references speak of its nature as drying, I have found that it does dry but also moistens. Because it has an effect on liver metabolism, it's possible that it balances tissue by drying excess water and bringing up oil, much like sage. But that is all speculative.

Uses:

- ➢ Historically used for damp/humid asthma; I have found it to be excellent for this, too.
- ➢ Chronic lung conditions
- ➢ Acute infections: bronchitis, pneumonia, colds, and flu
- ➢ Sinusitis with green discharge (though I have found it effective for yellow, as well)
- ➢ Parasitic infection

Sample Formulas:

- Bronchitis: tincture of elecampane, Solomon's seal, lobelia

- Cold: tincture of elecampane, calendula, ginger
- Sinusitis: tincture of elecampane, horseradish, osha, ginger, and cayenne (if ears are stopped up)
- Parasites: tincture of elecampane, black walnut hull, gentian root, fresh garlic (sliced clove swallowed whole), and eating pumpkin seeds

Eyebright (*Euphrasia canadensis*) - **Taste:** bitter, cool, dry. **Energetics:** astringent, anti-inflammatory. **Organ System Affinity:** nasal membranes, lungs, ears, eyes.

Contraindications: pregnancy, dry conditions
Part of plant used: above ground part of plant
Plant family: Orbanchaceae family
Used fresh, dried, or both: both
Best menstruums for extraction: water or alcohol
Medicine making dilutions: fresh plant tincture, 1:2; dried plant tincture, 1:5 (60% alcohol, 40% water); tea, ½ teaspoon of dried herb steeped for 10 minutes
Dosage: tincture, 3-4 drops; tea, 1-2 cups per day

According to Maude Grieve, eyebright is a Greek plant, with the name *Euphrasia* being derived from the word *Euphrosyne* meaning 'gladness.' She also says that in the 14th century, it was noted to "clear all evils from the eye."

Uses:

- Eyebright has few uses, as it is such a powerful astringent. Here are some of the times I don't use it, which are as important to be aware of as the times that you will use this plant. Do not use eyebright if: the nose is stuffy and congested, runny nose with a dry cough, dry mouth, or throat is dry with a runny nose.
- *Do* use it as a compress for inflammation of the eye with mucous and/or watery secretions, for conjunctivitis.
- Allergies with runny, wet secretions
- Sinusitis with lots of wet secretions

Sample Formulas:

- Sinusitis: tincture of osha, elecampane, echinacea, horseradish, eyebright

- Allergies: tincture of nettle leaf, echinacea, horseradish, eyebright
- Eye compress: herb tea bag of eyebright with a pinch of fennel seeds and a few drops of goldenseal tincture (evaporate alcohol off with hot water or use glycerin tincture instead)

Garlic (*Allium sativum*) - **Taste**: pungent, aromatic, warming, moistening. **Energetics**: diaphoretic, circulatory stimulant, anti-bacterial, expectorant, respiratory stimulant, anti-parasitic, anti-viral, anti-bacterial, emmenagogue, diuretic. **Organ System Affinity:** stomach, lungs, respiratory tract (lower and upper), colon, small intestine, heart, circulatory system, and blood.

Contraindications: allergy to garlic and onions
Part of plant used: bulb
Plant family: Liliaceae (lily family)
Used fresh, dried, or both: I prefer fresh
Best menstruums for extraction: honey, water, oil, alcohol, and vinegar
Medicine making dilutions: fresh plant tincture, honey, vinegar, or syrup, 1:2
Dosage: 4 tablespoons of garlic syrup per day or 20-30 drops of fresh plant tincture 3-4 times daily

Garlic has been in use as a food and medicine for thousands of years. In Ancient Egypt, those who built the pyramids to impart strength and vitality ate it with onion. According to Maude Grieve, the name garlic is Anglo Saxon and is reflective of the plant's leaf. *Gar-* 'a spear,' and *lac-* 'a plant.'

Uses:

➢ Garlic may be used topically to prevent infection, be it bacterial or viral (staph infections included). Simply cut a clove in half and apply the inner part of the clove to the cut.
➢ As an anti-bacterial ear oil. Please refer to Chapter 8 for specifics on how to use it.
➢ Culpeper recommends it for all cold diseases. That means, simply, to use garlic anytime cold is the root of the problem – acute infections, poor circulation, and low blood pressure with cold extremities.
➢ Garlic is great for heart health. It can reduce systolic and diastolic numbers by 5-10%; it lowers serum lipids, expands

vessel walls, decreases platelet aggregation (the tendency of red blood cells to clump together), and it may reduce cholesterol by 8% or more.

➢ As a great digestive tonic for those who struggle with parasites, candida, and intestinal bacterial infections.

Sample Formulas:

• Digestive health for parasites, bacterial infection, or candida: Take it with your favorite bitter so it won't hurt your stomach. I recommend gentian or *Angelica archangelica*. For 1-2 weeks, take 5 drops of the chosen bitter with meals. This primes the digestive tract. When ready, begin with the raw garlic. You will take your bitters, slice the clove, and then swallow said clove in the morning and in the evening before bed. Do this for a few weeks. There is also the option of the garlic fast, but that's far more intense.

• Ear infection formula: infused oil formulas of garlic, passionflower, and mullein flower oil or St. John's wort oil

• Heart health: Follow the instructions for digestive health, or use a tincture of garlic, ginger, hawthorn, and skullcap.

• Respiratory infections, croup, colds, and bronchitis: formula 1 - garlic with thyme syrup; formula 2 - garlic, thyme, ginger, elderberry syrup

Ginger rhizome (*Zingiber officinale*) - **Taste**: pungent, aromatic spicy, hot, dry. **Energetics**: vasodilator, anti-emetic, anti-coagulant, diaphoretic, anti-viral, digestive stimulant, carminative, cholagogue, anti-inflammatory, anti-spasmodic, expectorant, emmenagogue, for diarrhea and constipation, circulatory stimulant. **Organ System Affinity**: blood and circulatory system, digestive tract, respiratory tract, liver, uterus, immune system, heart.

Contraindications: should not be used regularly by those on blood thinners; avoid in large amounts in those with autoimmune disease, as their blood is already hot. Ginger can also speed the absorption of prescription or other drugs or medications, and should be taken hours after medications are ingested. Should not be used at all by those with a bleeding disorder.
Part of plant used: rhizome
Plant family: Zingiberaceae (ginger family)

Used fresh, dried, or both: both – fresh for circulatory disorders, colds and flus, constipation and digestive complaints; dried for digestion
Best menstruums for extraction: water, honey, and alcohol
Medicine making dilutions: fresh, 1:2; dried, 1:5 (60% alcohol, 40% water); I have also made a 1:1 tincture of fresh ginger.
Dosage: 1-2 tablespoons grated in 8 ounces boiled water, steep for 15 minutes, drink 1-3 cups daily; 5-20 drops of tincture 3-4 times daily

The name *Zingerber* is derived from Greek or Arabic and translates as 'known already to the Ancients.' This is reflected in the fact that it was first documented as a medicine in China around 4 B.C. The plant is also grown for its flower, which is fragrant and exquisite.

Uses:

> ➤ Is an excellent tea for colds and flus. The plant is drying and warming, an excellent expectorant and diaphoretic, and helps to stimulate the immune system.
> ➤ Circulatory conditions where cold hands and feet occur regularly
> ➤ Bronchitis that is in a wet and mucous heavy stage. There are times in bronchitis where the lungs feel hot and dry. If they do, don't use ginger! See Chapter 8 for more details on this.
> ➤ Inflammation of the joints when exacerbated by cold. You may use ginger topically as an infused oil or drink the tea regularly.
> ➤ Nausea, motion sickness, or morning sickness. Some contraindicate ginger with pregnancy, so check with your health care provider for further opinion.
> ➤ Ginger is an excellent anti-inflammatory and analgesic for headaches exacerbated by cold, sinusitis, or poor circulation.
> ➤ Ginger improves fat digestion by assisting the conversion of cholesterol into bile acids. It's also an excellent carminative that combines well with bitters and helps relieve either constipation or diarrhea.
> ➤ For low blood pressure with poor circulation
> ➤ For menstrual cramps (often accompanied with the inability of the period to begin) and intestinal cramps that improve

with pressure and warmth. May be used topically and drunk as a tea.

Sample Formulas:

- Colds: as a hot toddy tea of ginger, lemon, and honey; tincture of elderberry, ginger, echinacea
- Poor circulation: tincture formula of ginger and prickly ash
- Joint inflammation: infused oils of ginger, garlic, turmeric, rosemary, clove, with eucalyptus, clove and rosemary essential oils; internal tincture of ginger, turmeric, burdock root, nettle seed
- Nausea or vomiting: small sips of tea, or taking the powder internally
- Poor digestion: tincture of ginger, culvers root, gentian root, dandelion root
- Low blood pressure with poor circulation: tincture of ginger, hawthorn, collinsonia (if hemorrhoids with water retention in the midriff); tea of nettle leaf and ginger

Goldenseal *(Hydrastis canadensis)* - **Taste:** bitter, cool, stimulating, and drying. **Energetics:** anti-catarrhal, anti-microbial, anti-bacterial, anti-fungal, laxative, emmenagogue, cholagogue, cell regenerative (especially in the colon), astringent, muscular stimulant, mucosal anti-inflammatory and mucous membrane tonic, digestive tonic, increases production of hydrochloric acid. **Organ System Affinity:** mucous membranes, colon, stomach, sinuses, urinary tract, liver, bladder, uterus, immune system.

Contraindications: Excessive and long term use may interfere with vitamin B absorption (don't use for longer than 2-3 weeks); pregnancy, diabetes, nursing, high blood pressure
Part of plant used: root and rhizome
Plant family: Ranunculaceae (buttercup family)
Used fresh, dried, or both: both
Best menstruums for extraction: alcohol or oil (makes an excellent topical medicine when infused)
Medicine making dilutions: fresh tincture, 1:2; dried tincture or infused oil, 1:5 (60% alcohol, 40% water)
Dosage: 3-10 drops 3-4 times daily

Hydrastis is a North American plant that has become endangered. It grows in woods, and I have seen stunning stands of it in protected areas of the Appalachian Mountains. The root is a yellow to golden hue, which is how it comes by the name goldenseal. It is also known as *yellow root*.

According to Maude Grieve, the genus name *Hydrastis* is a combination of two Greek words – 'water' and 'accomplish.' She feels this is reflective of the plant's affinity for mucous membranes. It possibly is, as goldenseal is an effective mucous membrane tonic.

There have been many attempts to use other berberine rich plants in place of goldenseal. Oregon grape root (tinctured fresh) and yerba mansa (a southwestern plant) are two that I have tried. In truth, they are only marginally successful in replacing goldenseal. Yerba mansa I love for sinusitis and gastrointestinal infections, and Oregon grape root for gastrointestinal issues, but neither are true substitutes. In the words of Rico Cech, "There is no direct substitute for true cultivated goldenseal, which contains a unique array of isoquinoline alkaloids, is respected worldwide and occupies a special place in the hearts of American herbalists."

Note: please, use sparingly. Goldenseal is endangered, and, thankfully, quite potent in small doses.

Uses:

> ➢ This plant's ability to tonify and heal mucous membranes as well as create an environment that doesn't support infection is a part of its success.
> ➢ Sinusitis with yellow mucous
> ➢ Peptic ulcers and colitis
> ➢ Appetite stimulant
> ➢ Shigellosis
> ➢ Effective against protozoa, bacterial infections (strep included), and fungi
> ➢ Inefficient bile production resulting in hepatic (liver) congestion
> ➢ Chronic constipation
> ➢ Topically: eczema (wet only), ringworm, earaches, conjunctivitis

<u>Sample Formulas:</u>

- Topical for wet eczema: infused oil of goldenseal and plantain with essential oils of geranium and balsam peru
- Sinusitis (wet with yellow secretions): tincture of goldenseal, horseradish, echinacea, and osha
- Shigellosis: tincture of echinacea and goldenseal with peppermint
- Strep: tincture of echinacea, calendula, goldenseal, and poke root (topically, too)
- For pale and weak children prone to bacterial infections (this is an Eclectic doctor specific indication for goldenseal as a long term tonic): 1 drop of goldenseal 2-3 times daily
- Conjunctivitis: boil water, add 1 drop of goldenseal tincture and 2 drops of eyebright tincture to 1 tablespoon of boiling water to evaporate the alcohol off; use as eye drops 4 times daily

Holy basil (*Ocimum sanctum*) - **Taste:** aromatic, pungent, sweet, warming. **Energetics:** diaphoretic, diuretic, adrenal adaptogen, digestive tonic, carminative, anti-bacterial (mild), anti-oxidant, anti-viral, expectorant, immune stimulant/modulator, anti-inflammatory, anesthetic, cell regenerating (improves the elasticity of skin and speeds healing). **Organ System Affinity**: immune, stomach, nervous system, adrenals, mind/head, lungs, skin, circulatory system, women's reproductive system.

Contraindications: none known
Part of plant used: leaves and flowering tops
Plant family: Lamiaceae (mint family)
Used fresh, dried, or both: fresh for tincturing, dried for tea
Best menstruums for extraction: alcohol, oil, water, or honey
Medicine making dilutions: fresh tincture, 1:2; for tea, add 1-2 teaspoons to 8 ounces of water and steep covered for 15 minutes. Note: Basil is an aromatic plant. It's volatile/aromatic oils will evaporate easily. Steep covered and do not boil the leaves.
Dosage: acute tincture, 5-15 drops 3-4 times daily; acute tea, 2-3 cups daily; tonic tincture, 5-10 drops 3-4 times daily

Revered by the Hindu for thousands of years, holy basil occupies nearly every home or yard in India, regardless of class. It is considered a sacred protector, much like white sage is in American Indian culture, and can be found on altars and in front of houses.

Uses:

> Considered a *panacea* or 'heal all' in India. It's used for coughs, fevers, colds, indigestion, asthma, and fatigue. If you consider its energetics, you can see that holy basil appears to be a full body tonic, endocrine system included.
> Useful tonic for high blood pressure where stress is the culprit. Also acts as a diuretic.
> Adrenal adaptogen that helps our body better adapt to and cope with stress. It helps restore adrenal function and balance cortisol production, whether low or high.
> In digestive formulas for its carminative effects
> Is an anti-oxidant and anti-inflammatory, with the capacity to stimulate cell regeneration and cell repair
> Due to its high eugenol content (from the chemical class phenylpropene, and commonly associated with clove oil), it can be used for toothaches and internally as an anesthetic.
> Improves the elasticity of skin and speeds healing
> In formulas for mental clarity and to reduce mental fog and a cluttered mind. It is helpful here for those suffering from exhaustion, adrenal fatigue, and those recovering from a drug or alcohol addiction (sugar and caffeine included).
> As an adaptogen during the day that can help rebalance sleep cycles at night

Sample Formulas:

- Cold tea for fever and cough: holy basil, ginger, thyme
- Digestive aid: simple tea or tincture of holy basil with peppermint; tincture for the person who runs cold of holy basil, *Angelica archangelica*, yellowdock root
- Hypo thyroid support: tincture of holy basil, blue vervain, skullcap, and gotu kola or black walnut hull
- Daytime tincture for recovering drug or stimulant addict: holy basil, Siberian ginseng, yellow dock root, skullcap; or if anxiety is a daytime problem, holy basil, hawthorn, skullcap, motherwort

- Asthma support: tincture of huang qin, holy basil, nettle leaf (unless allergic), dandelion root or turmeric root
- General adaptogen formula: tincture of holy basil and skullcap

Horseradish (*Armoracia rusticana*) - **Taste:** pungent, slightly bitter, heating, thinning fluid, and slightly drying. **Energetics:** anti-oxidant, gut protective, expectorant, decongestant, bronchodilator, diaphoretic, anti-spasmodic, immune stimulant that raises white blood cell count. **Organ System Affinity:** stomach, sinuses, lungs.

> **Contraindications**: none known, but I avoid it with those who have thin hot blood and bleeding conditions, for this plant will heat the blood.
> **Part of plant used**: root
> **Plant family**: Brassicaceae (mustard family)
> **Used fresh, dried, or both**: fresh
> **Best menstruums for extraction**: honey and alcohol
> **Medicine making dilutions**: fresh plant tincture or infused honey, 1:2
> **Dosage**: used mainly in formulas – tincture, 2-5 drops 3-4 times daily; honey, ½ teaspoon 3-5 times daily

Uses:

➤ According to Maude Grieve, this root was used as a condiment to protect the gut from meat that was potentially bad (think food poisoning)
➤ Bronchitis when in need of a bronchodilator (also consider coffee)
➤ Sinusitis in formulas
➤ Internally for ear infections with sinus pressure and congestion
➤ Postnasal drip
➤ Food poisoning

Sample Formulas:

- Postnasal drip (wetness): honey or tincture of horseradish with tea of sage
- Food poisoning: tincture of horseradish and blue vervain

- Sinusitis: tincture of horseradish, elecampane, osha, echinacea; tea of 1 tablespoon of honey infused osha, elecampane, and horseradish in 8 ounces of hot water
- Ear infection: tincture of cayenne, horseradish, calendula, usnea, cleavers

Licorice (*Glycyerrhiza glabra*) - **Taste:** pungent, aromatic, sweet, slightly bitter, warm, and balancing to tissue (not too dry, not too moist). **Energetics:** demulcent, emollient, anti-spasmodic, diaphoretic, expectorant, anti-viral, laxative, antacid, adaptogen. **Organ System Affinity:** adrenals, sinuses, lungs, kidney, stomach, colon, liver, skin (topically).

Contraindications: high blood pressure, and not for long-term use
Part of plant used: root
Plant family: Fabaceae (legume family)
Used fresh, dried, or both: both
Best menstruums for extraction: best if tinctured in alcohol or macerated in oil; may use as a tea, but will not have the resins
Medicine making dilutions: fresh tincture, 1:2; dried tincture, 1:5 (70% alcohol, 30% water); tea, ½ teaspoon in 6 ounces of hot water
Dosage: Use for up to 3 weeks internally, 3-10 drops 3-4 times daily; 2-3 cups of tea daily

Glycyerrhiza is of the Greek word *glukurrhiza*, meaning 'sweet root.'

Uses:

➢ An anti-viral, expectorant, demulcent (from the resins), diaphoretic, and anti-spasmodic for acute respiratory infections such as bronchitis, pneumonia, and croup.
➢ Diaphoretic and anti-viral for general colds and flus
➢ Laxative for constipation but not for long-term use
➢ For ulcers or reflux with a bacterial affliction of the stomach; is antacid, anti-inflammatory and vulnerary (promotes wound healing, in this case, ulcers)
➢ An adaptogen that specifically acts as an adrenal cortex tonic when under-functioning
➢ Demulcent and emollient, but due to resins, which are alcohol and oil soluble (different from mucilaginous demulcent and emollient plants, which are water soluble)

> Potent anti-inflammatory with steroidal effects (both internally and externally). Great for chronic skin inflammation, psoriasis, and eczema when the infused oil is used in creams

> As an anti-diuretic with hypotension and frequent urination. It is specific for those who urinate clear urine in copious amounts.

> Surgical menopause over age 35 with *Angelica sinensis* (Michael Moore)

> According to David Winston, it "strengthens the adrenals, ovaries, hypothalamus, Isles of Langerhans." He recommends its use in autoimmune disease, but I don't typically use it for autoimmune conditions unless it is specific to the person. And even then, not for more than 3 weeks on and 3 weeks off.

Sample Formulas:

- Bronchitis: tincture of licorice, elecampane, lobelia; or tincture of licorice, Solomon seal, *Angelica archangelica*, lobelia
- As an anti-diuretic: tincture of licorice, agrimony, and yarrow
- External for psoriasis or eczema: infused oil of comfrey, licorice, calendula; if the condition is very dry, however, marshmallow root soaks
- Ulcers with acid reflux: tincture of licorice, chamomile, catnip, fennel; tea of licorice, fennel, and chamomile between meals
- Laxative for short-term use: tincture of licorice, dandelion root, fennel (if too dry) or caraway (if too wet), culvers root (if very poor fat digestion)

Linden (*Tilea spp.*) - **Taste:** sweet to acrid, for heat and wind. **Energetics:** diaphoretic, nervine and heart tonic, sedative, cephalic for headaches of high heat (of or relating to the head, here, drawing heat from the head downward), anti-inflammatory, hypotensive (when nervous), anti-spasmodic, mild demulcent/emollient and mild astringent (balances the tone of tissue). **Organ System Affinity:** nervous system, heart, blood and circulatory system, head, colon.

Contraindications: low blood pressure
Part of plant used: flowers and leaves
Plant family: Malvaceae (mallow family)
Used fresh, dried, or both: both
Best menstruums for extraction: water or alcohol
Medicine making dilutions: fresh tincture, 1:2; dried tincture, 1:5 (60% alcohol, 40% water); tea, 1-2 teaspoons per 8 ounces hot water steeped 10 minutes covered (to prevent volatile oils from escaping)
Dosage: 3-10 drops of tincture 3-4 times daily; 1-2 cups of tea daily

This tree, with its heart shaped leaves and fragrant flowers that apprehend to liberate the mind and what stress distracts it, is also called Basswood. It has two opposing properties, as it is considered a relaxant and stimulant. I don't see that as unusual, for many acrid plants that have effects on wind relieve constriction by relaxing the nervous system, and thereby stimulate circulation. I see linden as being similar. Also note that blue vervain is the same.

Uses:

> ➢ Nervous system agitation with insomnia
> ➢ Fevers with an inability to sweat and agitation
> ➢ Vertigo from stress or virus
> ➢ Nervousness and anxiety with high blood pressure
> ➢ Epilepsy
> ➢ Nervous diarrhea, as a nervine and demulcent with some astringent properties (to balance the tone of the colon)
> ➢ Influenza with fever

Sample Formulas:

- High wind constricted fevers: tea of linden blossom, yarrow, and catnip; tincture of blue vervain, linden, and yarrow
- Heart stress with anxiety: tea of linden, hawthorn; tincture of the same with motherwort
- Insomnia: tincture of linden, motherwort, passionflower
- Vertigo from stress: tea of linden, passionflower, and hawthorn berries; tincture of linden, passionflower, gingko, or hawthorn
- Vertigo from virus: tea of linden, hawthorn berries, and ginger root; tincture of linden, echinacea, and hawthorn

- Epilepsy formula: tincture of passionflower, lavender, and linden
- Diarrhea from nerves: tea of linden and catnip or of linden and fennel (if moistening is needed); tincture of linden, catnip (or fennel), and yellow dock root
- The flu: tincture of linden and yarrow; tea of the same

Lobelia *(Lobelia inflate)* - **Taste:** acrid, relaxing. **Energetics:** anti-spasmodic, expectorant, relaxing diaphoretic, emetic, anti-asthmatic, circulatory stimulant (due to its relaxant effect). **Organ System Affinity:** lungs, intestinal tract, heart, musculoskeletal system.

Contraindications: not for use in large doses, as it can be a powerful emetic

Part of plant used: leaves, stems, and seeds, harvested when in green seed pod stage (according to Richo Cech)
Plant family: Campanulaceae (bellflower family)
Used fresh, dried, or both: fresh or dried for tincture, dried for tea
Best menstruums for extraction: alcohol or water, but I prefer to use the tincture, as it is easier to gage your dose, and you don't want to take too much.
Medicine making dilutions: fresh tincture, 1:5 (75% alcohol, 25% apple cider vinegar, ACV)
Dosage: 2-10 drops 3-5 times daily

According to Maude Grieve, lobelia was named after the botanist Matthias de Lobel of London, who died in 1616.

Uses:

- Potent ant-spasmodic to the lungs, an indispensible formula plant for bronchitis, pleurisy, pertussis (whopping cough), croup, asthma. It is excellent and specifically used in the recuperative phase of these acute respiratory infections as well.
- Cardio anti-spasmodic specific for pains in angina
- Michael Moore says to use it in convulsive hysteria. I haven't done that yet, as I typically reach for passionflower here, but

I believe, since it is a relaxant to the nervous system, that it would be an excellent plant for such.
➢ Used by the Thomsonian practitioners to purge (make one vomit) the system as a prelude to a healing process. (I believe we've moved past that.)
➢ Works well as a liniment on bruises and sprains
➢ For intestinal colic
➢ An anti-convulsive used for epilepsy to reduce the frequency and number of episodes. I have not used it for this, but typically reach for passionflower or lavender.

Sample Formulas:

- Lower respiratory infections with high fever and dry, hot cough: tincture of lobelia, elecampane, Solomon seal, yarrow, and blue vervain; tea of marshmallow root
- Lower respiratory infections with lower grade fever and damp cough: tincture of lobelia, osha, ginger, and elderberry

Marshmallow root (*Althea officinalis*) - **Taste**: sweet, salty, cool, moistening/mucilaginous. **Energetics**: vulnerary (promotes wound healing), anthilithic (prevents formation of kidney stones), powerful demulcent, anti-inflammatory, cooling and moistening expectorant, anti-spasmodic, moistening laxative (not from stimulating peristalsis), diuretic. **Organ System Affinity**: lungs, intestinal tract, urinary tract, tissue, blood, immune system.

Contraindications: if a person has too much cold or moisture; should not be taken at the same time other medications or other herbs are ingested, because the mucilaginous quality can interfere with absorption. Allow an hour between.
Part of plant used: root, but sometimes the leaves (though the leaves are not as effective)
Plant family: Malvaceae family
Used fresh, dried, or both: dried
Best menstruums for extraction: water for the full mucilaginous effect; alcohol extraction is diuretic and anti-inflammatory
Medicine making dilutions: tea, 1:5 long cold infusion. Add your dried roots to water in a mason jar, cover and shake. Let sit for 6-8 hours/overnight, strain, and your infusion is ready.
Dosage: 2-4 ounces 4-6 times a day

Althea is of the Greek word *altho*, which means 'to cure.' Marshmallow root was seen as an effective healing remedy, as well illustrated by Pliny, the great philosopher, who believed if you took a spoon of water extract daily it would protect you from illness.

The plant grows 3-4 feet high and has 3-inch oval leaves that are soft and fuzzy. The flowers are like all mallow flowers, having unified stamens, taking on a kidney shape.

Uses:

> Soothing to all mucous membranes, so specific for dry respiratory infections, like the dry and hot natured bronchitis
> Perfect for croup, where the irritation and swelling is life threatening, and it has the ability to sooth the irritated larynx and throat
> Irritations of the intestinal tract with dryness and dry hard stools with constipation
> Urinary tract infections with inflammation, irritation, and burning
> Eczema and psoriasis that is dry and hot (internal consumption as well as external soaks). It will cool the blood, and move heat out from the skin, cooling and moistening the cellular matrix and immune system.
> Brings balance to extreme conditions. The mucilaginous coats the area in distress, softening the tissue and restoring water content in the cells. This doesn't merely affect the dryness but also decreases inflammation and acts as an anti-spasmodic and expectorant.
> Laryngitis of a hot and dry nature
> Post nasal drip with a dry throat
> Poultice for hemorrhoids
> A small amount in a hand cream is an excellent emollient for hot, dry, irritated skin. Think about the skin of winter (with infused oil of plantain or comfrey).
> Thought to have some blood sugar lowering effect, though I have not used it for such.

Milky oat seed *(Avena sativa)* - **Taste**: sweet, moistening, nourishing, and calming. **Energetics**: nervine tonic, anti-anxiety, stimulant, mild anti-spasmodic, anti-inflammatory, useful for weaning from addictive substances, nutritive to joints (oat straw). **Organ System Affinity**: joints (oat straw), nervous system, head.

160

Contraindications: gluten intolerance in some
Part of plant used: fresh milky oats
Plant family: Poaceae (grass family)
Used fresh, dried, or both: Fresh milky oat seed must be fresh; oat straw is used dried.
Best menstruums for extraction: milky oat seed is tinctured in alcohol; oat straw is made as a tea in water
Medicine making dilutions: fresh tincture, 1:2; tea of oat straw, 1-3 teaspoons per 8 ounces hot water steeped for 10 minutes
Dosage: 5-10 drops 3-5 times daily; 1-3 cups of tea daily

Uses:

➤ Milky oat seed tincture is sweet and specific for the dry, hot, and withered constitution. When someone has burned out as a result of too many life excesses or is feeling frayed and fried, milky oat seed tincture is a gift. Examples of a few of these excesses are: adrenaline stress, insomnia from stress, alcohol, caffeine, drugs, nicotine, late nights, taking care of the infirmed.

➤ It is specific for folks who have trouble focusing, insomnia from nervous exhaustion, headaches that radiate down the spine and into the lower extremities, impotence in men, swollen prostrate, PMS with exhaustion, and panic and epilepsy.

➤ Milky oat tincture was historically used to help wean from caffeine, drugs, and nicotine. I have had great experience using it for such as well. Two clients benefited from its effects who were cocaine abusers. They used the milky oat seed tincture after post withdrawal in a formula with adaptogens.

➤ Milky oats is an excellent nervine tonic for those debilitated by chronic pain, such as with arthritis and rheumatism. Oat straw tea is also very beneficial for joint health. It strengthens connective tissue weakness (hair, skin, nails), is nutritious, and specific for arthritis and complaints of the joints.

Sample Formulas:

• Insomnia: tincture of oats, passionflower, skullcap

161

- Nervine daytime formula: tincture of oats and St. John's wort
- Withdrawal from nicotine: tincture of oats, lobelia, elecampane, mullein leaf
- Heart health formula: tincture of oats, hawthorn, passionflower
- Daytime adaptogenic formula: tincture of oats, schisandra, hawthorn

Motherwort (*Leonurus cardiaca*) - **Taste**: bitter, acrid, aromatic, relaxing to nervous system and heart, stimulating to liver. **Energetics**: anti-spasmodic (heart, large intestine, uterus), anti-anxiety, nervine tonic, vasodilator, hypotensive, cardio tonic, emmenagogue, cholagogue (seeds), mild diuretic. **Organ System Affinity**: heart, Central Nervous System, uterus, large intestines/colon.

Contraindications: some high blood pressure medications; tincture is contraindicated in first 2 ½ trimesters of pregnancy
Part of plant used: flowering tops and leaves (without stems)
Plant family: Lamiaceae (mint family)
Used fresh, dried, or both: both
Best menstruums for extraction: alcohol, water, honey, and oil (though good luck getting someone to drink that bitter tea!)
Medicine making dilutions: fresh plant tincture, 1:2; dried plant tincture, 1:5 (75% alcohol, 25% water); tea, 1 teaspoon steeped 10 minutes in hot water
Dosage: tincture, 3-15 drops 3-6 times daily; 2 cups of tea daily

The Greeks gave motherwort the name 'mother's herb,' using the tea for pregnant women with anxiety. The tincture is often used in an Eclectic remedy, called Mothers Cordial. It is used the last 2-3 weeks of pregnancy to help prepare the emotional and physical body for birth. *Leonurus* is another Greek derived word. *Leon* means 'lion,' and *ourus* means 'tail.' When in flower, motherwort resembles a lion's tail. The species name, *cardiaca*, refers to 'heart,' for motherwort is a heart tonic.

While motherwort in flower looks like a lions tail, when I see motherwort in seed, I believe it looks like a spine. I find it a great medicine for people whose anxiety and nervousness prevent them from having one!

Uses:

> Motherwort encourages restfulness, is specifically a cardio (heart) and nervine tonic that improves mood. Maude Grieve describes the plant's action as follows: "There is no better herb for strengthening and gladdening the heart." It is true!
> While the tincture is contraindicated in the first 2 ½ trimesters of pregnancy, the tea is not, because the alkaloids that are emmenagogue and hypotensive are only alcohol soluble; therefore, the tea is fine. Beware, though, for it is very bitter!
> High blood pressure from stress and anxiety, especially when mood is affected.
> Nervous tachycardia, arrhythmias, and palpitations
> Improves blood density by decreasing clotting factor and lessening how much fat is in the blood.
> Premenstrual tension and syndrome
> Menstrual cramps and difficulty starting
> General anxiety in men and women
> Anxiety and insomnia in those with hyperthyroidism (including autoimmune)
> Autoimmune disease where stress and anxiety triggers a disease flare
> Central Nervous System sensitivity and agitation

Sample Formulas:

- Anxiety: daytime tincture of motherwort, hawthorn, skullcap; nighttime tincture of motherwort and passionflower, or motherwort and blue vervain
- Heart palpitations with low blood pressure: tincture of motherwort, hawthorn and rosemary; with high blood pressure, motherwort, hawthorn, and passionflower or garlic
- General insomnia: tincture of motherwort, passionflower, California poppy
- PMS with anxiety, dysmenorrhea (menstrual cramps): tincture of motherwort, skullcap and ginger (ginger if cramps respond positively to warmth, and there is difficultly beginning bleeding)
- Hyperthyroidism: tincture of motherwort, passionflower, lemon balm, and bugleweed (only 5 ml of bugleweed in a 30 ml bottle)

Osha (*Ligusticum porterii*) - **Taste:** pungent, aromatic bitter, carrot like flavor, oily, warm, and drying. **Energetics:** diaphoretic, anti-spasmodic, anti-bacterial, expectorant, decongestant, bronchial dilator, emmenagogue, carminative, mild anti-histamine, anesthetic to mucous membranes. **Organ System Affinity:** sinuses, lungs, stomach, uterus, skin.

Contraindications: pregnancy and dry conditions, as it is quite drying
Part of plant used: root
Plant family: Apiaceae (parsley/carrot family)
Used fresh, dried, or both: both
Best menstruums for extraction: alcohol or water
Medicine making dilutions: fresh tincture, 1:2; dried tincture, 1:5 (70% alcohol, 30% water); 1 teaspoon simmered for 30 minutes in 6 ounces of water. Note: When the root tincture is finished macerating in alcohol, I pour the tincture off, take the un-pressed roots that are still holding tincture and infuse them in honey for a week or two. I then use this infusion with the root to make tea. I do this with most of my roots, but my favorites are elecampane, horseradish, ginger, and osha.
Dosage: tincture, 5-15 drops 3-5 times daily; tea, 1-3 cups daily

Uses:

> Influenza, colds, and lower respiratory infections that are irritated and mostly dry
> Head colds and sinusitis with headaches, moisture, sore throat, and irritation
> Allergies
> Respiratory infections that are wet
> Back when I participated in sweat lodges, both in Kentucky and in New Mexico, osha tea was one of the herbs poured over the hot stones inside the tent. I find, to this day, that an osha bath is a beautiful thing if becoming ill. When the bathroom is steamy, you steep in the tea and inhale the vapors.
> Used by the Cochiti Indians of the Southwest in a salve for cuts, bruises, and irritations. They also used a paste of the root powder to draw out poisons from venomous spider, snake, and insect bites.

Sample Formulas: (See *Elecampane* for sample formulas.)

Passionflower (*Passiflora incarnata*) - **Taste:** sweet, acrid, relaxing. **Energetics**: sedative, anti-emetic, anti-anxiety, anti-spasmodic, anti-convulsant, hypotensive, anti-histamine, anti-arrhythmic, analgesic, anti-psychotic, anti-brandykinin. **Organ System Affinity**: nervous system, heart, hypothalamus, respiratory.

Contraindications: use with anti-depressant drugs, anti-anxiety medications, benzodiazepines; use with caution with high blood pressure medications.
Part of plant used: of the vine, stems, flowers, and leaves
Plant family: Passifloraceae (passionflower family)
Used fresh, dried, or both: both
Best menstruums for extraction: water or alcohol
Medicine making dilutions: fresh plant tincture, 1:2; dried plant tincture, 1:5 (60% alcohol, 40% water); tea, 1 teaspoon-1 tablespoon steeped in 8 ounces of hot water for 1 minute
Dosage: tincture, 2-10 drops 2-4 times daily; tea, 1-2 cups daily

Uses:

➢ Lung anti-spasmodic specific for asthma
➢ Muscle relaxant for tightness (includes heart)
➢ According to the Eclectic doctor King, it is specific for hypertension with elevated diastole and palpitations.
➢ Anxiety with insomnia
➢ PMS with insomnia, anxiety, and uterine heaviness
➢ According to Michael Moore, it is specific for hypertension with tinnitus (ear ringing) and headaches. I have used it in formulas for this with good success.
➢ Migraine in the evenings from low blood sugar
➢ Hysteria from psychoactive drugs
➢ Hyperthyroidism with bulging eyes
➢ Anti-spasmodic for nervous system disorders (heart pain, headaches, menstrual cramps, neuralgia)
➢ Anti-convulsant for Parkinson's and epilepsy
➢ High fevers with insomnia, agitation, and/or disturbing dreams and waking visions
➢ Decreases heart rate while raising respiratory rate and neuromuscular action

> Prevents brandykinin and histamine reaction in the allergic response (brandykinin is a polypeptide that plays a role in allergic inflammation, similar to histamine response)
> Potent sedative that produces a narcotic effect
> High in the flavonoids courmarin and carborylic acid (at their peak when flowering)
> Mexican uses: childbirth, blood tonic, social drink, fruit as a food (John Muir said it was the most delicious fruit); root topically for boils, hemorrhoids, earaches

Sample Formulas:

- Insomnia: tincture of passion flower, Californica poppy, motherwort (if anxiety)
- Parkinson's: tincture and tea of skullcap and passionflower
- High fever with bad dreams and hallucinations: tincture of passionflower, yarrow, and blue vervain; tea of passionflower, catnip, and yarrow
- PMS with heavy uterus and cramps: tincture of passionflower and motherwort
- Hypertension (for starters): tincture of hawthorn, passionflower

Peppermint (*Mentha piperita*) - **Taste:** pungent, aromatic, slightly sweet (if the flowers are used with the leaves), warms to cool, and drying. **Energetics:** anesthetic, anti-inflammatory, anti-spasmodic, carminative, anti-emetic, cholagogue, nervine, slightly astringent, mild immune stimulant. **Organ System Affinity:** head/brain, respiratory tract (sinuses and lungs), stomach, large intestines, liver, nervous system, mild affinity for the circulatory system, immune system.

> **Contraindications**: epilepsy; stomach ulcers and inflammatory conditions of the stomach or intestinal lining, especially when dryness is a part of the problem (peppermint is very drying)
> **Part of plant used**: flowering stalk with leaves (not woody stems); the flowers lend a sweetness to the pungent leaves and make an amazing tincture that is far less irritating as the leaves alone.
> **Plant family:** Lamiaceae (mint family)
> **Used fresh, dried, or both:** both, but dried mint should not be more than 6-8 months old and should be stored away from

light and heat; it is high in volatile oils that are age, light, and heat sensitive (yes, all mints are).
Best menstruums for extraction: water, alcohol, honey, and oil.
Medicine making dilutions: fresh tincture, 1:2; dried tincture in oil or honey, 1:5 (75% alcohol, 25% water); tea, add 1-2 teaspoons to 8 ounces of hot water, steep covered for about 5-10 minutes.
Dosage: tincture, 2-5 drops 3-4 times daily; tea, 1-3 cups daily

The name *Mentha* comes from Mintha, a Greek nymph. There are many stories that illustrate how Mintha became the mint plant, but the one I am most familiar with says that Mintha, in a fit of jealousy and rage at the loss of her lover to another, was stepped on by Demeter, and there grew as a mint plant.

Robert Tisserand, the aromatherapist, tells a slightly different tale in his book, *The Art of Aromatherapy*. "Mint was once the nymph Mentha, whom Pluto found extremely attractive. Persephone, his jealous wife, pursued Mentha and trod her ferociously into the ground! Pluto then changed Mentha into a delightful herb."

The species name, *piperita*, literally translates as 'pepper scented mint.'

Most people don't know, but peppermint is a hybrid of water mint and spearmint. It hybridized itself in the wild hundreds of years ago. So the mint referred to as *Mentha* above is actually water mint or spearmint. Which? I can't remember.

Uses:

> ➢ Intestinal viruses: it is anti-emetic and anti-nausea, which is great for those suffering. The anesthetic, anti-spasmodic, carminative, and anti-inflammatory aspects come in handy here as well, lessening irritation and that which is driving the virus to be unbearable.
> ➢ Headaches especially resulting from digestive distress, heat, or stress.
> ➢ Allergies! The French have found peppermint to be a benefit to allergies. It lessens the effect of histamine on tissue and reduces histamine production in the liver.

➢ Peppermint is an excellent formula plant for those with chronic disease of the gallbladder and pancreas where poor bile production interferes with digestion. Increases bile production in liver and stimulates release from gallbladder; reduces inflammation and spasms.
➢ Poor digestion with fermentation, gas, low intestinal bowel flora
➢ Sinusitis: peppermint penetrates mucous membranes, thinning and drying mucous. It also helps relieve headaches that result.
➢ Colds with wet runny noses.

Sample Formulas:

- Allergies, if wet and runny: tea of peppermint with tincture of nettle leaf, peppermint leaf, eyebright, and osha
- Sinusitis: tincture of peppermint, elecampane, echinacea, horseradish; tea of ginger and peppermint
- Cold: tea of peppermint, ginger, osha root, and yarrow; if recurrent, add tincture of peppermint, echinacea, and osha
- Digestive tonic for chronic gastritis: tincture of cinnamon, peppermint, dandelion root
- Nervous stomach: tea of peppermint, lemon balm, catnip
- Stomach virus: tincture of peppermint, blue vervain, and anise hyssop; tea of peppermint and catnip with honey
- Gallbladder insufficiency: tincture of peppermint, culvers root, dandelion root or artichoke leaf; tea of peppermint and fennel
- Headache: tincture of St. John's wort, peppermint, willow bark, blue vervain; tea of peppermint, lavender

Plantain leaf (*Plantago major*) - **Taste:** salty, mucilaginous, cooling, and drying. **Energetics:** astringent, anti-septic, mild alterative, diuretic, styptic, drawing agent, demulcent, emollient, speeds cellular regeneration in mucous membranes, vulnerary (wound healing) that heals from the inside out (unlike comfrey, which heals from the outside in), anti-inflammatory, expectorant, mild anti-spasmodic. **Organ System Affinity:** lungs, stomach, large intestine, skin, bladder, vagina (topical).

Contraindications: where there is a dry external chronic condition; on abscesses where a styptic is inappropriate, for one does not want to stop the flow of fluid, even blood

168

Part of plant used: leaves
Plant family: Plantaginaceae (plantain family)
Used fresh, dried, or both: both
Best menstruums for extraction: water for the mucilage, or alcohol for other constituents
Medicine making dilutions: fresh tincture, 1:2; dried tincture, 1:5 (75% alcohol, 25% water); tea, 1 teaspoon steeped in 8 ounces hot water for 10 minutes; poultice, 1 teaspoon leaf moistened and applied to affected area
Dosage: tincture, 5-10 drops 3-4 times daily; tea, 1-2 cups daily

The name, *Plantago*, translates from two Latin words, *planta*, meaning 'sole,' and *ago*, meaning 'like.' It was thought that plantain resembled the sole of a shoe.

Uses:

➢ Rich in chlorophyll and high in allantoin (which speeds cellular regeneration)
➢ Ulcers of the stomach or colon to speed healing and decrease inflammation and irritation
➢ Respiratory infections with lots of irritation
➢ Coughs where the lungs feel hot and dry
➢ Cystitis with mucous in the urine and irritation
➢ Diarrhea with colon irritation
➢ Eye inflammation with irritation (use tea as drops)
➢ For bug bites and stings (chew the fresh leaf and apply topically as soon as possible. It loses its potency if you wait)
➢ According to Culpepper, plantain is an excellent plant for high hot heat resulting in a headache. He wasn't alone. It is well noted that New Mexicans did a similar thing, binding the leaves to the forehead to remove heat and relieve the headache.
➢ For gout and rheumatism
➢ As a leaf poultice for tooth aches, or an infused oil for earaches

Sample Formulas:

• Coughs: tea of plantain with other supporting herbs (see Chapter 8, *Plants for Acute Respiratory Infections*)
• Gout and rheumatism: tea of burdock root, plantain, dandelion root

- Eye drops: tea of fennel, eyebright, and plantain
- Cystitis: tea of plantain and yarrow; tincture of uva ursi with yarrow
- Ulcers: as a tea of plantain with chamomile, drunk between meals

Sage (*Salvia officinalis*) - **Taste:** pungent aromatic, warm, brings up oil, and dries water. **Energetics:** diaphoretic, carminative, astringent, anti-bacterial, anti-viral, anti-oxidant, anti-inflammatory, anti-galactagogue, cholagogue, emmenagogue. **Organ System Affinity:** stomach, immune system, hormonal/milk ducts, lungs, sinuses, lymph glands, liver.

Contraindications: pregnant or nursing
Part of plant used: leaves and flowers
Plant family: Lamiaceae (mint family)
Used fresh, dried, or both: both
Best menstruums for extraction: water, honey, alcohol or oil (use dried for the oil)
Medicine making dilutions: fresh tincture, 1:2; dried tincture, 1:5 (75% alcohol, 25% water); tea, 1 teaspoon steeped in 8 ounces of hot water covered for 10 minutes
Dosage: tincture, 5-10 drops 3-4 times daily; tea, 1-2 cups daily

Maude Grieve tells us that *Salvia* comes from the Latin word *salvere*, 'to be saved,' but I have learned the translation may also mean 'whole' or 'sound.'

Uses:

➢ As a hot tea for colds with profuse runny nose and wet cough
➢ Laryngitis with excess nasal secretions
➢ Gargle for sore throat, tonsillitis, and laryngitis
➢ Drink sage tea or take the capsules of sage to wean from nursing. It will dry up your milk (sage dries moisture). You can make your own capsules by purchasing sage in the cooking herb section and unfilled capsules in your local health food store. Yes, it works powerfully well for this.
➢ Used topically as an infused oil for abscesses
➢ As a hair rinse for alopecia
➢ Specific indications for sage as a tonic from the Eclectic physician, Dr. John King (practiced in KY in the late 1800's):

skin has relaxed, is moist, circulation poor with cold, copious amounts of sweat

<u>Sample Formulas:</u>

- Cold and flu, for wet runny conditions: tea of sage, ginger, osha
- Hot flash formula: tincture of sage, motherwort, kava
- Abscess salve (for drawing out infection): sage and St. John's wort infused oil, essential oil of clove and lavender, tincture of yerba mansa or pine, blood root, echinacea (see Chapter 10 for more on how to work with abscesses)

Skullcap leaf (*Scutellaria lateriflora*) - **Taste**: bitter, pungent, cooling, and drying. **Energetics**: Central and Autonomic Nervous System tonic/adaptogen, nervous system anti-spasmodic (for respiratory, heart, tremors and ticks in Parkinson's, mild Tourette's, and restless leg), cholagogue. **Organ System Affinity:** Central and Autonomic Nervous System, liver, stomach, lungs, heart.

Contraindications: none known
Part of plant used: flowering tops (without stems)
Plant family: Lamiaceae (mint family)
Used fresh, dried, or both: most effective fresh; if dried, not more than 6-8 months old
Best menstruums for extraction: alcohol or water
Medicine making dilutions: fresh plant tincture, 1:2; dried plant tincture, 1:5 (60% alcohol, 40% water); tea, 1 teaspoon-1 tablespoon per 8 ounces of hot water steeped and covered for 10 minutes
Dosage: tincture, 2-10 drops 3-4 times daily; tea, 1-2 cups daily

<u>Uses:</u>

- Anti-spasmodic for stomach, heart, respiratory tract (when ANS is the trigger)
- Mild cholagogue
- Tremors and ticks in Parkinson's, mild Tourette's, and restless leg
- Spastic cough during a cold or flu that does not respond to anti-spasmodics; the cough is the result of a nervous tick and responds beautifully to skullcap, an Autonomic Nervous System anti-spasmodic.

- ➢ Anxiety and nervousness
- ➢ Nervous conditions with hand or body tremors
- ➢ Performance anxiety for sports, musicians, actors, and speakers
- ➢ Anxiety and adrenaline that raises blood pressure
- ➢ Headaches with nervousness and anxiety
- ➢ Autoimmune conditions
- ➢ Digestive disorders and Irritable Bowel Syndrome

Sample Formulas:

- Anti-spasmodic to lungs with a cold: catnip, skullcap, elecampane (if mucous)
- Anxiety and nervousness with stomach issues: tincture of skullcap, peppermint, and yellow dock root or dandelion root; tea of skullcap and lemon balm
- High blood pressure from adrenaline stress and performance anxiety: tincture of motherwort, skullcap, hawthorn (may also add milky oat tincture or holy basil)
- Headaches from nervousness and anxiety: tincture of skullcap, peppermint, and blue vervain; tea of skullcap and peppermint
- Headaches from fat digestion with nervousness: tincture of skullcap, artichoke leaf, ginger rhizome
- Autoimmune disease with anxiety and stress: tincture of skullcap, blue vervain, hawthorn

Thyme (*Thymus vulgaris*) - **Taste:** pungent, aromatic, herbaceous, warm, stimulating to immunity but relaxing to tissue, thereby penetrating and loosening. **Energetics:** expectorant, anti-viral, anti-bacterial, anti-fungal, carminative, anti-oxidant, anti-spasmodic, diaphoretic, emmenagogue, diffusive organ. **Organ System Affinity:** lungs, stomach, immune system, mucous membranes, skin.

Contraindications: none known
Part of plant used: flowers with leaves
Plant family: Lamiaceae (mint family)
Used fresh, dried, or both: both
Best menstruums for extraction: water, honey, alcohol, or oil

Medicine making dilutions: fresh tincture, 1:2; dried tincture, 1:5 (75% alcohol, 25% water); tea, 1-2 teaspoons steeped in 8 ounces of hot water covered for 10 minutes
Dosage: tincture, 3-10 drops 3-4 times daily; tea, 1-2 cups daily

The name thyme has an interesting origin, and people don't necessarily agree what the name means. In some circles, I have heard that it is derived from the Greek word *thumus*, meaning 'courage.' Maude Grieve makes note of this origin as well as another. That the word thyme translates as 'to fumigate.' Seeing as the plant was recognized for its pleasing scent but also for its stimulating effect, it's probable that both translations are correct.

Uses:

> Culpepper says it is a "noble strengthener of the lungs."
> I have used it successfully in formulas for damp coughs and for dry coughs.
> An exceptional plant in formulas for RSV, whooping cough, bronchitis, and pneumonia. It combines especially well with garlic for these illnesses. You may also use thyme for symptom relief with antibiotics.
> Colds, flus, and respiratory illnesses with stuck and stagnant mucous. It loosens thick mucus and relieves congestion, as it is penetrating. While it is warming, it is diffusive, meaning it helps to move heat.
> Intestinal spasms and general gastrointestinal problems. It has been historically viewed as having a strong affinity for the gastrointestinal tract when there is spasm, gas, colic, bloating, poor digestion, and elimination.
> Topically, thyme as an infused oil or essential oil is an excellent remedy for fungal infections, rheumatic and joint pain, sprains and strains.

Sample Formulas:

• Topical pain and inflammation: thyme and sage infused oil rub with essential oils of eucalyptus, lavender and clove
• Wet coughs: tincture of osha, thyme, elecampane, wild cherry bark
• Dry coughs: syrup of garlic, thyme; tincture of thyme, elecampane, Solomon seal, lobelia

- General gastrointestinal distress: tea of thyme, peppermint, holy basil

Usnea (*Usnea barbata*) - **Taste:** acrid, relaxant, warm. **Energetics:** potent anti-bacterial and anti-fungal, anti-spasmodic, pharyngeal mucosal tonic, mucilaginous (water soluble). **Organ System Affinity:** immune system, lungs, large intestine, skin, bladder, mouth, mucous membranes.

> **Contraindications**: highly irritating to the stomach, so use in small doses
> **Part of plant used**: whole plant
> **Plant family:** Parmeliaceae (lichen family)
> **Used fresh, dried, or both:** dried
> **Best menstruums for extraction:** alcohol (95% product); if the mucilage is needed, soak in water overnight.
> **Medicine making dilutions:** dried plant tincture, 1:5 (70% alcohol, 30% water)
> **Dosage:** 3-5 drops 4-5 times daily; with bacterial infections, take for 2-3 weeks

Usnea, the plant commonly referred to as 'old man's beard,' was branded so due to its appearance. It looks like a beard. Usnea grows all over the world, with its use as a medicine dating back 3,000 years in China.

Usnea is part fungus and part lichen.

Uses:

> ➢ Usnea, being anti-bacterial and mucilaginous, gives it bragging rights amongst herbs. It's an unusual combination. Dr. Rudolph Weiss says of usnea and its relative medicinal lichens, "The action of lichens appear to be similar to those of the ribbed plantain, except that the anti-bacterial effect is more marked in their case."
> ➢ The moistened plant may be used as a wound dressing, topically on skin abrasions to prevent infection and as a bandage. It may also be applied to boils and abscesses to help soften and open the wound.
> ➢ Its anti-fungal properties give it potency as a topical medicine as well. Using the tincture of infused oil in a salve on eczema, ringworm, and fungal infections. I find that fungus or bacteria often find their way into long or short

standing outbreaks of eczema and psoriasis. Usnea is an excellent plant, topically and internally here.
➢ Internally for Candida or fungal infections of the respiratory tract and vagina
➢ Internally for bacterial infections of the respiratory tract. It is effective against staphylococcus, pneumonia, whooping cough, and bronchitis (rarely bacterial, though). It is safe to use in small doses with antibiotics to help the body better fight the infection.
➢ For cystitis, as it is an excellent anti-bacterial that is less irritating than uva ursi
➢ A mouth rinse for mouth infections or inflammations

Sample Formulas:

- Strep throat: tincture of usnea, calendula, poke root, echinacea, cleavers
- Cystitis: tincture of usnea, yarrow, corn silk
- Ring worm: salve of calendula infused oil; tincture of usnea and echinacea, essential oils of balsam peru, clove, geranium, cardamom
- Eczema and Psoriasis: tincture of usnea, burdock root, cleavers; topical (if tolerated) infused oils of calendula; tincture of usnea, black walnut hull, licorice (or infused oil); essential oil of balsam peru and geranium
- Respiratory infection from fungal infection: tincture of usnea, calendula, echinacea, cardamom (if wet)

Yarrow flower (*Achillea millefolium*) - **Taste:** bitter, pungent, acrid, calms tissue, slightly astringent. **Energetics:** anti-inflammatory, anti-spasmodic (to smooth muscles), anti-oxidant, anti-diarrheal, anti-septic, anti-viral, styptic, diaphoretic. **Organ System Affinity:** urinary, nerves, blood, liver, smooth muscles.

Contraindications: allergy to aspirin, beware
Part of plant used: flowering tops with leaves, no woody stems
Plant family: Asteraceae (compositea/sunflower family)
Used fresh, dried, or both: both
Best menstruums for extraction: alcohol, oil, water, and honey

Medicine making dilutions: fresh tincture, 1:2; dried tincture, 1:5 (75% alcohol, 30 % water); tea, 1-2 teaspoons of herb steeped in 8 ounces of hot water for 10 minutes
Dosage: 5-10 drops of tincture 3-4 times daily; 1-2 cups of tea daily

Achillea millefolium, the Latin name for yarrow, defines a part of mythology as well as the physical plant structure. *Millefolium* is derived from *milfoil*, meaning 'million-leaved plant.' This refers to the many segments of its foliage. *Achillea* is derived from the warrior, Achilles, who is said to have used it to stop the bleeding wounds of his soldiers. As a result, warriors have carried yarrow into battle for centuries for its healing power and the spirit of courage and protection the plant brings to those who wear it.

The common name, yarrow, is derived from the Dutch and Saxon words *gearwe* and *yerw*. In the herb world, it is said that *gearwe* means 'healer.' The term *gearwe* is also used in many Old English stories in the context of war. To translate loosely, *gearwe,* in the *Anglo-Saxon Dictionary of Weapons*, is defined as 'to arm oneself in some way,' be it protective clothing or wrapping weapons for battle. This makes reference to the spiritual use of yarrow for protection.

Uses:

> ➢ Excellent remedy for colds and flus, as it relieves aches, reduces discomfort from sore throats, dries a wet runny nose, pains and reduces fevers, including high ones!
> ➢ Yarrow is anti-inflammatory for several reasons: the chemical constituents salicylic acid, (which is shares with willow and meadow sweet) and azuline (a relative to one of chamomile's main anti-inflammatory constituents, chamazuline). It is also high in flavonoids, which stimulate the body to produce prostaglandins that control smooth muscle contractions. So not only does yarrow decrease inflammation, it is also a decent anti-spasmodic.
> ➢ In formulas for menstrual cramps when there is too much bleeding (do not use if you need an agent to stimulate bleeding)
> ➢ For postpartum bleeding in case of hemorrhage
> ➢ Anti-inflammatory to bladder and bowel
> ➢ Urinary tract tonic post infection (anti-inflammatory and anti-septic)

➢ For urinary tract infections, especially when blood is present
➢ Stops bleeding from deep wounds, works in less than a minute.
➢ The anti-inflammatory and astringent effects make yarrow effective for varicose veins, piles, and to help lower blood pressure.

Sample Formulas:

- Postpartum bleeding or hemorrhage: tincture of yarrow, shepherds purse, cramp bark or motherwort. Take 30-60 drops of tincture of the combined plants every 20-60 minutes until bleeding stops or danger has passed.
- Headaches: tincture of yarrow, feverfew, blue vervain
- A bath to stop bleeding: yarrow tea or tincture with the tincture of St. John's wort and calendula. Soak or baste area for 5-10 minutes.
- Urinary tract infections: tincture of yarrow, usnea, uva ursi; tea of yarrow, corn silk (organic only), and marshmallow root (see marshmallow root for the proper way to use this plant)
- Urinary tract infections, post infection: tea of yarrow, parsley, and burdock root
- High fevers: tincture of yarrow, catnip, and blue vervain: tea of linden and yarrow

Chapter 12

Infused Oil Materia medica

Many plants that we infuse in oils to use topically have specific internal uses, too. While this chapter focuses solely on external use, you will find the following plants from this chapter in Chapter 11, Internal Plant Medicines *Materia medica*: calendula, mullein, plantain, and sage.

Arnica (*Arnica montana*): Arnica is warming, a potent anti-inflammatory, and increases small capillary circulation where applied. The capillary stimulation shuffles out toxins that build up in an injured and inflamed area, while also stimulating the body's innate ability to heal the wound. Arnica is specific for external injuries with bruising and swelling and should not be applied to broken skin. Where there is broken skin, I apply arnica around the area. It still works to lessen inflammation.

Specific Uses: arthritis, muscle strains, sprains, accident and sports/dance injuries, broken bones to decrease local swelling when the incident occurs, and where there is muscle soreness later. Combines very well to work synergistically with St. John's wort infused oil.

Calendula (*Calendula officinalis*): This infused oil is typically made with fresh flowers, but I have found dried to be just as effective if they are not older than one year. The oil is anti-fungal, anti-bacterial, anti-inflammatory, anodyne, a mild styptic, anti-oxidant (aiding cell repair), and an excellent lymphatic. It is also very high in Vitamin A. Calendula oil and tincture are both safe to use topically on deep wounds.

Specific Uses: bug bites, diaper rash, bacterial vaginitis, cervical dysplasia, cuts, scrapes, and irritations. It works beautifully with St. John's wort infused oil for punctures and deep gashes to lessen pain and keep tissue health so that infection does not set in.

Chaparral (*Larrea spp.*): This aromatic bushy shrub from the dessert is anti-oxidant, anti-inflammatory, anti-bacterial, and anti-fungal. I love the scent, which is oily, dusty, earthy, and aromatic. An all-purpose salve formula that I simply adore for scent as well as use is: chaparral infused oil with essential oils of myrrh, vetiver, frankincense, balsam peru and geranium.

Specific Uses: joint and bursa inflammation, irritated skin conditions, wound healing, sun burns, fungal infections, and as a topical anti-oxidant.

Comfrey root or leaf (*Symphytum officinale*): It's high in allantoin, which gives it the capacity to heal scratches, abrasions, minor burns, skin irritations, and regenerate broken bones very quickly. It is contraindicated on puncture wounds or any injury that goes beyond the surface of the skin, for it heals the outer dermal layer too quickly, encapsulating infection, and often leading to abscesses or causing the infection to move into the blood.

Warning: *Never use comfrey root internally. The leaf can be used in tea formulas for no longer than 2-4 weeks. To use comfrey to knit broken bones, I recommend taking the homeopathic.*

Specific Uses: skin irritations, bruising, sprains, minor burns

Mullein flower (*Verbascum thapsus*): This oil is a potent anti-inflammatory and anodyne.

Specific Uses: Most herbalists, myself included, use mullein flower oil for earaches. It combines well with garlic and St. John's wort infused oil to help fight infection and decrease pain. But I also find it useful for relaxing and realigning the spine, broken bones, hip injuries, and in formulas for sore muscles. In most of these cases, I will mix it with arnica infused oil or St. John's wort.

Plantain (*Plantago major*): Plantain is emollient, cell regenerating, cooling, drawing, and slightly drying. It contains the same chemical constituent that comfrey has, allantoin. While comfrey heals from the outside, plantain heals from the inside. I still hesitate to use it on wounds that need to stay open to prevent infection, but I do find it useful after the threat of infection has passed.

Specific Uses: a drawing poultice with clay to draw out infection (must combine it with something warming if the infection is deep and with anti-bacterial plants), apply immediately to a spider bite, bug bite, or sting for best results. If time goes by, it is less effective.

Sage (*Salvia officinalis*): Sage is warming, astringent, dries moisture but brings oil up out of the skin, anti-microbial, stimulating, anti-inflammatory, and anti-oxidant (just like many of its kitchen garden companions). Sage infused oil is one for moist skin that lacks oil and is therefore slightly dry but damp.

Specific Uses: abscesses, for damp skin in creams and lotions, as an external anti-oxidant, in formulas for arthritis, muscle and bursitis inflammation, and sprains. For abscesses, use with St. John's wort infused oil and tinctures of myrrh, blood root, clove (or essential oil), and lavender. For joint and muscle pain, combine with arnica and calendula, with essential oils of eucalyptus, ginger, lavender, rosemary, and clove or cinnamon.

St. John's wort (*Hypericum perforatum*)**:** This is an anodyne (fast acting), nerve regenerator, anti-inflammatory, anti-viral, and anti-spasmodic. This plant is potent in very specific ways. It lends its medicine in consort with others harmoniously and also plays well solo. The thing to remember about St. John's wort infused oil is it stops pain within seconds to minutes of applying. That is no joke. Punctures, severe cuts, and deep gashes are all made to feel better by direct application of the oil or tincture of St. John's wort. It also assists nerve regeneration when they are severed.

Specific Uses: sprains, bruises, and external swellings of all kinds, deep cuts, punctures, abscesses (with other more specific plants), spasms, sciatica (external and internal). For use on swellings, sprains, and bruises, combine with comfrey and arnica infused oil, tincture of blue vervain (assists the blood being reabsorbed into the blood stream, thereby decreasing swelling), and eucalyptus and lavender pure essential oils. For nerve regeneration on deep wounds, combine with calendula infused oil and tincture of echinacea.

Chapter 13

Essential Oil *Materia medica*

The essential oil *Materia medica* is organized differently than the internal plant chapter. Here is how you will see things laid out:

Common name (*Latin Name*) - **Scent, Energetics, Organ System Affinity**

Contraindications
Part of plant used (in distillation)
Plant family

Here you will find writing about the meaning of the name and history of the essential oil.

* Uses with Sample Formulas.

Cinnamon (*Cinnamomum zeylanicum*) - **Scent**: pungent and sweet. **Energetics**: warm, anti-bacterial, anti-inflammatory, anti-viral, anti-fungal, anesthetic, nervous system and circulatory stimulant, warm and dry expectorant. **Organ System Affinity**: blood, circulatory system, nervous system, respiratory tract, immune system, muscles and joints.

Contraindications: sun exposure, sensitive skin
Part of plant used: leaf or bark (I recommend using the leaf; it's far less irritating)
Plant family: Lauraceae

Cinnamomum zeylanicum is a tall evergreen tree native to Sri Lanka. Its history as a healer begins before Christ. The name *Cinnamomum* is of the Greek, *kinnamomon*. It is thought to translate from the Phoenician as 'sweet wood.' But there is some indication that it may also mean 'pipe like,' in reference to the hollowness of the twigs. *Zeylanicum* is derived from the name *Ceylon*, which was Sri Lanka's original name.

In Ancient Egypt, cinnamon was used in formulas for its warming properties. It raised the temperature of the body, thus stimulating circulation and the nervous system, counteracting fatigue and depression. It was added in topical preparations for the stomach, in poultices to relieve muscle and joint pain, and in Holy Oils and burning rituals. Cinnamon was also used in the aromatic oil formula for mummification. The body was rubbed with juniper oil, after which the abdominal cavity was filled with cinnamon and myrrh as a preservative and for their fragrant odors.

Uses with Sample Formulas:
- Cinnamon stimulates the nervous system, mind, and the respiratory tract. Sample topical formula for such uses: cinnamon, rosemary, peppermint, and frankincense. It can be inhaled or rubbed at the temples and on the legs.

- It is a warming anti-inflammatory for muscles and joints, a circulatory stimulant to relieve emotional pain associated with physical pain, and is an anesthetic. Sample formula to be used topically in a salve: clove, rosemary or eucalyptus, lavender, cinnamon, and peppermint (if you like).

- Cinnamon is an anti-bacterial. As an inhalation it can be used for strep throat, pneumonia, meningitis, or staphylococcus. It warms and stimulates the blood and immune system, while having broad reaching anti-bacterial effects. Sample formula: lavender, cinnamon, thyme, and marjoram. For strep, add 1 drop of cinnamon pure essential oil to a teaspoon of water and gargle for a minute 1-3 times daily to numb pain and act as an anti-bacterial.

- It is excellent when used in hospital settings where the risk of a complicating respiratory infection is high due to immune impairment. I especially love cinnamon in conditions where the complication of a lower respiratory bacterial infection would be life threatening. Examples of this are adults or children undergoing cancer treatments, those with HIV or AIDS, and the elderly. I recommend putting a drop on a cotton ball and setting it by the bed or putting it in the pillow. Foot rubs with diluted oils are also specifically indicated here.

- Use drops of essential oil in a cold water humidifier for acute respiratory infections, upper or lower. Sample formula: cinnamon, lavender, spikenard or marjoram, and *Eucalyptus globulus*. A salve of this formula applied to the feet and chest of the person is essential support, too, and will help control a cough (for more on this, see Chapter 8, Herbs for Acute Respiratory Infection).

Clary Sage (*Salvia sclarea*) - **Scent**: sweet, floral, woody. **Energetics**: warm, dries moisture in skin but brings up oil, anti-anxiety, sedative, nervine tonic, hypo-tensive, mild anti-fungal, anti-spasmodic, anti-inflammatory, aphrodisiac, astringent, emmenagogue. **Organ System Affinity**: uterus, nervous system, head.

Contraindications: breast cancer, first 2 ½ trimesters of pregnancy, and sometimes epilepsy
Part of plant used: leaves and flowers
Plant family: Lamiaceae

Salvia sclarea is a species of sage that is native to Europe and has become a beautiful and hardy addition to American gardens. It grows tall, sometimes up to six feet and has large thick and hairy green leaves.

Salvia is a genus that has between 700 and 900 different species. It translates as 'whole' or 'sound.' The species name, *sclarea,* is a reference to the 'sclera' or white of the eye, denoting that the seeds were once used as a wash to clear eye obstruction, redness, and inflammation.

If you have ever grown clary sage, and I highly recommend it, you know that working and being around it is an intoxicating and joyous experience. Perhaps the Germans figured this out, as they once made beer from this plant.

Uses with Sample Formulas:

- Clary sage is excellent support for those who are stressed, anxious, have insomnia, and nervous debility. Sample formulas for baths, massage, or body oils: lavender, bergamot, and clary sage; clary sage, rosewood, eucalyptus; ylang ylang, clary sage, and mandarin; lavender, lemongrass, clary sage.

- Clary sage is known to have some estrogen like effects due to the high sclearol content. When a woman's cycle is short, meaning less than 28 days from day 1 of one period to day 1 of the next period, clary sage may be an excellent ally for them. But women without short cycles may use clary sage also. It may specifically be used as an emmenagogue for PMS headaches or for menstrual cramps. Cramp oil should be applied topically over the uterus, for painful spasms, and to bring on menstruation if it is delayed. A sample formula: clary sage, ginger, and lavender in arnica infused oil.

- Clary sage is an excellent aphrodisiac for women who lose interest in sex due to hormonal imbalances, the physical process of pregnancy, a hysterectomy, or menopause. Sample formulas for support are: rosewood, ylang ylang, ginger, and clary sage, or cinnamon, clary sage, and mandarin.

- While contraindicated during pregnancy due to its action as an emmenagogue, clary sage makes an excellent tonic for the two weeks before the due date. When used in small amounts during this time (a .5% dilution), it has the ability to prepare the body for what is to come physically, emotionally, and chemically. It warms a cold and fearful constricted womb and relaxes the nerves to inspire labor. I find it specific for women with high blood pressure and the inability to achieve active labor due to the fear of birth and motherhood. My favorite formula for birth preparation simulates labor, the respiratory tract, relaxes the nerves, and helps with mental clarity. It is also anti-anxiety. The formula is: rosewood or rose, clary sage, cardamom, and *Eucalyptus globulus*. Another formula that I have successfully used to bring on active labor and calm the anxious laborer is lavender, clary sage, and grapefruit. These formulas may also be used post-birth to help rebalance hormones and to calm the nerves and spirit.

Eucalyptus _(Eucalyptus globulus)_ - **Scent**: pungent, menthol based, slightly sweet. **Energetics**: cools to warm, analgesic, anti-inflammatory, mild anti-bacterial, respiratory anti-spasmodic, decongestant, and a drying expectorant. **Organ System Affinity**: lungs, sinuses, head, circulatory system.

Contraindications: urinary tract infections, toxic internally, may be used in small dilutions topically, but I have seen it give a rash to sensitive pale skinned individuals
Part of plant used: leaves
Plant family: Myrtaceae

Eucalyptus is native to Australia but has been cultivated globally. It is a genus of plants with over 700 species. Jeanne Rose tells us that _Eucalyptus_ means 'well covered,' and is in reference to the calyx, which forms a lid over the flower. _Globulus_ translates as 'globe like.'

Uses with Sample Formulas:

• Eucalyptus can be used in formulas for acute upper and lower respiratory infections. It is anti-spasmodic, decongestant, and a stimulating expectorant. I recommend adding a few drops in a humidifier, to pots of hot water to steam up a room with scent, to a hot shower, or to a salve base (1% dilution) to be applied to the chest and feet. A few sample formulas are: lavender, marjoram, and eucalyptus; spikenard, cinnamon, lavender, eucalyptus.

• Eucalyptus can also be used for tension headaches. It cools to reduce inflammation and warm, thereby increasing circulatory power and lessening constriction from tension. It is also an analgesic, helping relieve nerve pain. Sample formulas can be applied in 1% dilutions to the temples, back of neck, inhaled for a few minutes. Formulas are: lavender, eucalyptus, ginger; lavender, clary sage, eucalyptus; lemon, lavender, chamomile, eucalyptus, and peppermint.

- Eucalyptus can reduce pain and inflammation from muscle strain, joint pain, and bursitis. Topical salves made as a 1% dilution do very well to manage symptoms of physical pain as well as emotional pain associated with chronic pain. Sample formulas: rosemary, clove, lavender, and eucalyptus; lemongrass, eucalyptus, frankincense or clove; peppermint, rosemary, lavender, and eucalyptus.

Frankincense (*Boswellia carterii*) - **Scent**: sweet, pungent, spicy. **Energetics**: warm, astringent, lymphatic tonic, expectorant, anti-spasmodic to the lungs, sedative, diuretic, anti-septic, nervine tonic, anti-inflammatory, anti-asthmatic. **Organ System Affinity**: immune system, nervous system, lymphatic system, lungs.

Contraindications: none known
Part of tree used: resin
Plant family: Burseraceae (torchwood family)

In Middle English and Old French, frankincense means 'high quality incense.' It was discovered thousands of years ago in the land now called Somalia. The tree thrives in an astonishingly stark and harsh environment, growing where the land is dry and barren, and it produces a fragrant resin rich in heritage.

Historically, symptoms that warranted the internal use of frankincense were ulcers, vomiting, tumors, dysentery, and fevers. Inhalations were used for respiratory infections, such as bronchitis and laryngitis. In Ancient China, frankincense was used for leprosy to quicken the blood, thereby stimulating circulation in blocked meridians and relieving pain.

Frankincense was used by the Egyptians to aid the release of the soul from the body in religious rituals. It facilitated their connection with the spirits and raised their level of consciousness. Frankincense was also used internally in preparations for physical and spiritual weakness.

It was often combined with cypress and cedar wood in a recipe for anointment. While the specific use of this formula is unknown, we can guess the purpose it served. Cypress and cedar wood are both oils for preservation and transition into the afterlife, with frankincense being for strength and protection to safely pass to the spirit world. So perhaps the trio of plants was for life and death transitions or evolutionary shifts of the soul and spirit.

Frankincense essential oil is widely used.

Uses with Sample Formulas:

- It can be used for the lungs as a foot application, healing bath, and inhalation. Formula: frankincense, clove, mandarin, cinnamon.

- Frankincense brings balance to a frayed nervous system. Use it in healing baths, in inhalations, or oils to rub on the feet. Excellent combinations for this are: lemongrass, frankincense, clary sage; mandarin, frankincense, clove; lavender, frankincense, cedar wood.

- Those with Post Traumatic Stress Disorder find solace with frankincense. It makes a person feel safe and centered where there was once chaos. It is a great plant ally when used in tandem with a therapist. Frankincense with talk therapy may more effectively help heal trauma. I also recommend making massage oils. Some formulas to try: frankincense, myrrh, mandarin; ylang ylang, frankincense, sweet orange, geranium; frankincense, bergamot, lavender.

- Grief comes in many forms and greatly affects the nervous system and lungs. A combination that reaches grief should be specific per person, for some people need warming, and some need cooling. A nice grief formula that warms is: clove, cinnamon, mandarin, and frankincense. A cooler and calmer formula for grief: peppermint, cypress, cedar wood, frankincense. A woody and neutral formula: rosewood, cedar wood, and frankincense.

- When eliminatory organs are taxed, and edema or varicose veins begin to set in, take a warm bath in frankincense, vetiver, small amounts of grapefruit, and cedar wood.

- To support and stimulate blood, immune, and lymphatic circulation when it is stagnant, causing swellings in lymph nodes, take a bath in, or rub the legs and midriff down with a 1% dilution of this formula: grapefruit, cypress, vetiver, and frankincense.

- Hemorrhoids: Apply this salve made as a 1% dilution to the affected area: St. John's wort and calendula infused oils, and essential oils of frankincense, vetiver, and lavender.

- Topical skin inflammation and irritations do well with frankincense. It is also specific for dry and aging skin. Use the essential oil in clay facials or in aqueous sprays for the face. You may want to combine it with lavender and vetiver pure essential oils.

- In general, I like to use healing baths to clear the energy field of a person. It's a general tool for preparing someone for spiritual healing work. Almost all plants are candidates for this work, but frankincense is specific for it, especially if trauma is great (such as PTSD, as mentioned previously). Fear and shock is moved to the side with this plant. People become more capable of connecting with and releasing pain with the regular use of frankincense. It makes them feel safe and lifts a soul depressed. This is a major step to getting perspective and setting a new healing and life course.

Geranium (*Pelargonium graveolens*) - **Scent**: sweet, floral, slightly pungent. **Energetics**: warming, analgesic, mild anti-bacterial and anti-viral, anti-septic, anti-fungal, balances the water and oil content of the skin, diuretic, stimulates adrenal cortex, emotionally sedative or balancing. **Organ System Affinity**: immune system, nervous system, skin, urinary tract, adrenals.

Contraindications: sun exposure
Part of plant used: leaf
Plant family: Geraniaceae

Uses with Sample Formulas:

- Geranium is an effective agent topically for fungal and bacterial infections. Skin infections are complex. When tissue is too moist or too dry, it's left prey to invading pathogens. If the condition goes untreated for a while or is unsuccessfully treated, other infections may also invade. This means that one will have a dual infection of a bacterial and fungal nature, or viral and fungal nature. Geranium is effective against infections but also brings balance to skin, inspiring oil production just enough to influence water content in sebaceous and sweat glands. It reduces inflammation when there is a red rash that is dry or flakey and moist.

I have used it on toddlers whose rash would not respond to other anti-fungal plants, such as myrrh and tea tree (both of which are too dry and astringent). A dilution of geranium alone cleared up the infections. It is also an essential oil in my ringworm formula. For ringworm (1-2% dilution): balsam peru, geranium, clove, cardamom, lavender, myrrh and small amounts of peppermint. Diaper rash or other rashes on a baby (.5% dilution): chamomile, geranium, and lavender in infused oil of calendula.

- As an anti-viral and cold and flu support, try a hand spray of geranium, lemongrass, thyme, and cinnamon. A bath formula of geranium, lavender, and lemongrass is nice, too.

- Geranium calms and balances the adrenals and nervous system. As with all nervine tonics that affect how the body uses energy, one might feel sedated at first, but after a few weeks, will notice that they have more energy. Formulas for nervous system balance: geranium, lavender, and lemongrass; or geranium, rosewood, and frankincense.

- To maximize the sedative effect and use geranium in formulas for insomnia, combine geranium with other sedatives. Sample formulas: clary sage, geranium, and mandarin; or geranium, lemongrass, and ylang ylang.

- For skin that lacks oil but is moist, there is still a dry quality to it. A cream or salve with geranium and clary sage will help with this problem.

- Geranium is anti-septic and diuretic. It is very useful for urinary tract infections and edema. For those going to the bathroom often but having little production, take a salt bath using geranium and yarrow pure essential oils. For chronic edema, use a bath or body oil of geranium, vetiver, cypress, and grapefruit (small amounts of grapefruit for the bath).

- Emotionally, I have used this oil on clients with Post Traumatic Stress and those who suffered from abuse. They are constantly reacting to the world around them. Geranium helps them remember a more emotionally balanced approach to life and decreases reactivity to stress. Some formula examples: geranium, frankincense, and mandarin; geranium, frankincense, and ylang ylang; geranium, grapefruit, and ylang ylang.

Lavender (*Lavandula angustifolia.*) - **Scent**: sweet, floral, pungent. **Energetics**: analgesic, anti-spasmodic, anti-septic, carminative, diaphoretic, cell regenerating, nervine, flu, spastic cough, headaches, appropriate for migraines, nervous tension, insomnia, muscle aches and pains. **Organ System Affinity:** immune system, skin, nervous system, muscles, digestive tract, respiratory tract.

Contraindications: internally with anti-coagulant drugs (lavender has blood thinning effects); wounds where there is heavy bleeding
Part of plant used: flowers
Plant family: Lamiaceae

Like many prolific plant medicines, lavender has been in use for over 2,500 years. Its Latin root, *lavare,* translates as 'to wash,' also lending itself to the term *lavatory,* meaning 'washroom.'

Lavender, itself, was historically used as a wash and was added to baths, cleaning fluids, and laundry tubs for its scent. Its scent was also widely used at the time of the Black Plague. To protect themselves from the plagues stench, people saturated their floors with lavender and wore bunches of flowers around their wrists and necks. It became known that towns who distilled lavender essential oil were virtually plague-free, as were grave robbers who washed their hands with an essential oil formula that had lavender in it, called 'Thieves Oil.'

Uses with Sample Formulas:

- Lavender makes a mild yet effective anti-microbial salve that is great for family use. The base of the salve is St. John's wort and calendula infused oils with a 1% dilution of lavender pure essential oil.

- You can also use lavender in a stronger anti-bacterial salve. The base of this would be calendula infused oil, with tinctures of echinacea and usnea, and pure essential oils of thyme, lavender, and geranium.

- As an analgesic for headaches, try one or more of these formulas: eucalyptus, peppermint, and lavender; bergamot, lavender, and clary sage; or lavender, peppermint, and ginger.

- Lavender is great in cold and flu formulas. It relaxes the nervous system, is diaphoretic, and also helps fight infection. For cold and flu formulas, choose 2 or 3 of the following oils: lavender, thyme, peppermint, eucalyptus, or cinnamon. For a spastic cough: lavender, sweet marjoram, thyme, and eucalyptus; or lavender, spikenard, and eucalyptus.

- Internally, when used as a tea or tincture, lavender is specific for digestive complaints with nervous tension and colic in infants. The plant can be inhaled to assist this problem as well. For adults, I combine it with peppermint and ginger for such times. You can simply inhale and apply it to the affected area. For infants, toddlers, and children, add 2 drops of lavender pure essential oil to olive oil and apply gently and slowly in clockwise circular motions to the belly. In some cases, this can also relieve constipation.

- Anti-anxiety: lavender, lemongrass; lavender, geranium, and lemongrass; ylang ylang, grapefruit, and lavender; frankincense, lavender, and bergamot; rose or rosewood, lavender, and balsam peru.

- Insomnia: Lavender outpaced benzodiazepines in sleep studies with the elderly. Not only did it work just as well, if not better, at getting folks to sleep, it improved mood throughout the day. Formulas for kids and adults of all ages can be applied to the feet or put on cotton balls inside pillows. A few examples: lavender, mandarin, and ylang

ylang; lavender, clary sage, and rose or geranium; lavender, mandarin, and spikenard; or simply use lavender alone!

- Nervous system imbalances do well with lavender. Try using a sleep formula of lavender with other complimentary essential oils applied to the feet (see insomnia formulas), and apply more enlivening oils during the day. Examples: lavender, frankincense, and peppermint; lavender and vetiver; lavender and cedar wood; lavender, petitgrain, sweet orange, and frankincense.

- Burns, both chemical and heat, are helped by lavender. There are many options for burn treatment. I've used lavender pure essential oil applied neat to small areas. I've also successfully used an oil of 1 ounce of St. John's wort infused oil and 6 drops of lavender pure essential oil successfully for chemical and radiation burns. Sunburns on adults and children do well with aloe vera gel and a few drops of lavender essential oil added. I've seen the reddest, nastiest burns be remedied overnight with the lavender and aloe vera formula.

- Cell regeneration: For a combination that is packed with skin cell regeneration properties, lavender and chamomile pure essential oils can be combined with rose hip seed oil and St. John's wort infused oil. Wound healing from deep cuts, gashes, or punctures: lavender and yarrow essential oil, St. John's wort and calendula infused oil, echinacea tincture (about 60 drops in 2 ounces of salve).

- Lavender is the grandmother, and I consider it to be a great plant for learning and remembering self-compassion. You have to admire a plant that comes from so deep in history to help the human spirit remember our plant allies, as it did when it connected with the French aromatherapist Gattefosse, a story noted in Chapter 2. It has the ability to relieve stress in the soul and slow down time to help us regain our balance, and to gather our strength in a moment of difficulty before pieces of us scatter. By retaining our wholeness, we live in the greatness of who we are; we are more capable of compassion and understanding.

Lemongrass (*Cymbopogon citratus*) - **Scent**: green and herbaceous, earthy, citrusy. **Energetics**: warm, nervine tonic, sedative, anti-anxiety, hypo-tensive, muscle relaxant/vasodilator, anti-infectious, anti-inflammatory, astringent for oily skin, anti-microbial, headaches. **Organ System Affinity**: heart, nervous system, skin, respiratory tract, immune system, lymphatic system, circulatory system.

Contraindications: none known, but use sparingly in incidence of hypotension (low blood pressure)
Part of plant used: leaves
Plant family: Poaceae

Lemongrass is native to India and China. It is used in medicine as a tincture, tea, essential oil, and in healing soups for respiratory infections.

Uses with Sample Formulas:

• Lemongrass as a remedy for anxiety is bold and effective, but gentle. It may be used for insomnia as a foot rub, in bath formulas, or inhaled. Sample formulas for anxiety or insomnia: lavender, petitgrain, and lemongrass; ylang ylang, mandarin, and lemongrass; clary sage, lemongrass, ylang ylang, and sweet orange. One of my favorite formulas for anxiety is a musical 'C chord,' as decided by G. W. Septimus Piesse, PhD, in his book, *The Art of Perfumery*. The formula is: lavender, lemongrass, and vetiver. This formula is a great emotional body harmonizer. It helps resynchronize the nervous system and rest of the body when anxiety has adversely affected someone.

• As a hypotensive, lemongrass is a vasodilator (substance that widens the blood vessels by relaxing the vessels muscular wall opposite of vasoconstriction). I have used it in formulas that support therapies for high blood pressure and tachycardia. For high blood pressure: clary sage, lemongrass, and lavender. Tachycardia: lemongrass with ylang ylang.

• Lemongrass relaxes muscles, thereby improving fluid transport, increasing circulation and all over body health. This is part of why this little plant can do so many things. When we decrease stress and tension, we improve health and function over all, even if the plant was not specific to the person. When good health cannot be attained in part because of stress and tension, use lemongrass! The relief provided allows us to observe our client better and define the true root of the problem.

- There are many performers and sportsmen out there who suffer from nervousness to the point where they turn to beta-blockers. This class of drug suppresses the effects of adrenaline on the heart, thereby reducing nervousness. I have successfully used an aromatherapy formula of ylang ylang, lemongrass, mandarin, and vetiver with supportive internal herbal therapies to balance the energy of the heart and make the effects of adrenaline more manageable. Hopefully, performers and sportsmen will begin to turn to these alternatives instead of this very harmful class of drugs.

- Lemongrass is a mild astringent and specific for oily skin when applied topically for clinical effects. It is also indicated for edema with cellulite. It tones skin structure and supports the elimination of excess water and toxins in the cells. One example of a formula for edema: grapefruit, frankincense, and lemongrass.

Mandarin (*Citrus reticulate*) - **Scent**: sweet and sour. **Energetics**: cooling, sedative, anti-anxiety, quiets the chatty mind, anti-viral, anti-microbial, astringent. **Organ System Affinity**: nervous system, heart, respiratory tract.

Contraindications: skin irritation if used in large amounts; allergy to citrus
Part of plant used: peel
Plant family: Rutaceae

Mandarin's Latin name, *Citrus reticulate*, translates as 'citrus with netlike membrane.' Anyone who has eaten a mandarin knows about this netlike structure that surrounds the ball of fruit under the peel.

All citrus oils have the following energetic actions to varying degrees: anti-microbial, anti-viral, and astringent. While mandarin is the least likely choice for use as an anti-viral and anti-microbial for it is not as strong as grapefruit or lemon, it is one I typically want in a sedative formula. Mandarin is unique. It is the only citrus fruit that contains a chemical constituent called anthranilic acid. Anthranilic acid is a powerful sedative, which makes mandarin an excellent choice when one is needed.

Uses with Sample Formulas:

- Mandarin has a strong synergy with other oils for insomnia. My favorite sleep formula: rose (can substitute geranium or rosewood), spikenard, and mandarin. You can also try lemongrass, mandarin, and lavender; or ylang ylang, mandarin, and clary sage. As instructed Chapter 9, apply the formula to the feet.

- Clinical anxiety is an excellent place for essential oils. Using inhalations and smelling salts throughout the day, one can help change a person's mind about their experience. Sample formulas are: mandarin, lemongrass, and clary sage; ylang ylang, mandarin, and frankincense; mandarin, grapefruit, and lemongrass.

- Citrus oils balance oily skin. One can use them in small amounts in clay facials or in bath and body oils. For a clay facial, add 1 drop each to a tablespoon of facial: mandarin, grapefruit, and lavender. Mix well and apply to the face. Let it sit for 10 minutes, then rinse. For bath and body oils, the same formula can be used in a 1% dilution. You might also try mandarin, cypress, and lavender; mandarin, cedar wood, and frankincense or geranium.

- Mandarin is not specifically recommended for irregular heartbeats, but can help. When the heart begins to beat to a different rhythm, anxiety can be exacerbating the problem. I include mandarin in formulas for irregular heartbeat for this reason. Try one of these formulas: mandarin, vetiver, and ylang ylang; lemongrass, mandarin, ylang ylang, and clary sage; frankincense, ylang ylang, and mandarin.

Vetiver (*Vetiveria zizanoides*) - **Scent**: pungent, earthy, slightly sweet. **Energetics**: cooling, aphrodisiac, lymphatic, strengthens circulation and a weakened immune system, repels insects, nervine tonic. **Organ System Affinity**: lymph, immune, nervous system.

Contraindications: none yet
Part of plant used: root
Plant family: Poaceae

Vetiver is a tall grass that grows in India. According to *Narong Chamchalow*, this quote from a Vetiver newsletter sums up the translation of the name: "Vetiver is originally a French word, derived from a Tamil word, *vettiveru* (*vetti* = to dig up, *ver* = root)."

The essential oil is a steam distillation of the root and is considered a panacea. When the root is harvested for distillation, the grass is woven into blinds that hang in the windows of houses in India to keep out the blaring sun. The essential oil, which is thought to have a cooling effect on the physical and emotional body, is then sprayed onto the grass blinds.

Uses with Sample Formulas:

- Aphrodisiac formulas are fun to come up with. Vetiver is an excellent earthy scent to compliment many of the other aphrodisiacs, which are spicy and sweet. Some suggestions: vetiver, mandarin, ylang ylang, and cinnamon; vetiver, clary sage, and mandarin; vetiver, geranium, and mandarin; clary sage, geranium, cardamom, and vetiver.

- Vetiver is an effective nervine tonic. It is a specific treatment for nervous system debility from too much emotional stress and deep-rooted tension and fears. If insomnia is an issue, a treatment plan should include a formula to balance the nervous system during the day and one that is sedative for night. Daytime formulas may be: vetiver, lavender, and lemongrass; vetiver, geranium (or rosewood), cedar wood, and cinnamon; vetiver, frankincense, cinnamon, and cedar wood. Nighttime formulas: mandarin, vetiver, and lavender; vetiver, ylang ylang, and clary sage; vetiver, geranium or rosewood, and mandarin.

- Vetiver combines well with warming oils to help strengthen the immune system. Formulate specific per person, for immune deficiency affects people in many different ways. Some general suggestions: vetiver, frankincense, thyme, and cinnamon; vetiver, lavender, and lemon; or thyme, clove, and vetiver.

196

- Those who get frequent swellings in the lymph glands need lymphatic tonics. Bathing and massage can help. Coupled with a regular application of a supportive essential oil formula and an internal herbal formula, swellings can be greatly decreased in size and frequency. Some essential oil formulas that may be used as a general application, bath oil, or massage oil (make as 1% dilution): vetiver, cypress, and frankincense; vetiver, grapefruit, and cypress; frankincense and vetiver.

- Insect repellants are made to be mass marketed, but according to many studies, they aren't always effective. The reason is that plants work to repel insects by interacting with a person's natural scent. This meeting of plant scents and human pheromones is what repels insects. That means, not one repellant will work for all. Keep that in mind when formulating your repellant. There are many plants to choose from here, such as patchouli, vetiver, lavender, basil, thyme, clove, cinnamon, peppermint, and catnip. Sample formulas: clove, vetiver, lavender, and geranium; or catnip, peppermint, lavender, basil, and clove.

- Cooling foot sprays are satisfying on hot summer days. For information on how to make the spray, please refer to Chapter 7. Formula examples: lavender, vetiver, peppermint, and eucalyptus; geranium, vet iver, and peppermint.

Ylang ylang (*Cananga odorata*) - **Scent:** fruity, floral, sweet. **Energetics:** anti-septic, aphrodisiac, hypo-tensive, sedative, anti-anxiety, cardio tonic, (specific for heart palpitations as it regulates cardiac rhythm), calming nervine tonic, euphoric, frigidity, aphrodisiac for impotence, sedative for insomnia, oily skin. **Organ System Affinity:** nervous system, heart, respiratory tract, reproductive system.

Contraindications: none yet, but may cause headaches if over used
Part of plant used: flowers
Plant family: Anonaceae

Ylang ylang is known as 'the poor person's jasmine.' Its common name translates from the Tagalog, *ilang ilang*, to 'flower of flowers.' Its Latin name, *odorata*, means 'scented.'

Ylang ylang's flower has an undeniable effect on the heart and nervous system, as it posses the ability to normalize an abnormally fast heart beat and slow rapid breathing. It came to be extensively used by Dr. Jean Valnet, a French physician, who successfully used essential oils to treat soldiers with PTSD and wrote the book, *The Practice of Aromatherapy* based on his experience.

Uses with Sample Formulas:

- Formulas to regulate cardiac rhythm: lavender, lemongrass, and ylang ylang; clary sage, ylang ylang, and lemongrass; grapefruit, lavender, and ylang ylang.

- Palpitations with rapid breathing: ylang ylang, lemongrass, and frankincense.

- High blood pressure: ylang ylang, clary sage, and grapefruit; geranium, ylang ylang, and clary sage.

- Aphrodisiac (for play and frigidity): geranium, vetiver, and ylang ylang; ylang ylang, cinnamon, ginger, and vetiver; clary sage, mandarin, and ylang ylang; ylang ylang, mandarin, and geranium or rosewood.

- Ylang ylang is anti-anxiety and is a mental pacifier for chronic frustration and anger. Sample formulas: lemongrass, ylang ylang, and clary sage; geranium (or rosewood), ylang ylang, and cedar wood; mandarin, ylang ylang, grapefruit, and lavender; ylang ylang, vetiver, and cedar wood.

Bibliography

Cech, R. (2000). *Making Plant Medicine*. Williams, OR, USA: Horizon Herbs Publication.

David M.R. Culbreth, P. M. (1927). *A Manual of Materia Medica and Pharmacology*. Philadelphia, PA, USA: Lea and Febiger.

Grieve, M. (1971). *A Modern Herbal* (Vol. 1). (L. Mrs. C.F, Ed.) New York , NY, USA: Dover Publishing, Inc.

Grieve, M. (1971). *A Modern Herbal* (Vol. 2). (M. C. Leyel, Ed.) New York, NY, USA: Dover Publishing, Inc.

Jean Valnet, M. (1982). *The Practice of Aromatherapy*. (R. Tisserand, Ed., & L. C.W. Daniel Compant, Trans.) Rochester, VT, USA: Healing Arts Press.

John William Fyfe, M. (1903). *The Essentials of Materia Medica and Theraputics*. Cincinnati, OH, USA: The Scudder Brothers Company.

Mary Bove, N. (1996). *An Encyclopedia of Natural Healing for Children and Infants*. New Canaan, CT, USA: Keats Publishing, Inc.

Moore, M. (2003). *Medicinal Plants of the Mountain West*. (M. Wachs, Ed.) Santa Fe, NM, USA: Museum of New Mexico Press.

Pengelly, A. (1996). *The Constituents of Medicinal Plants*. Merriwa, New South Wales, Australia: Sunflower Herbals.

Rudolf Fritz Weiss, M. (1985). *Herbal Medicine* (6th German edition ed.). (F. M. A.R. Meuss, Trans.) New York, USA: Thieme.

Tisserand, R. B. (1977). *The Art of Aromatherapy*. Rochester , VT, USA: Healing Arts Press.

W.M. H. Cook, M. (1869). *The Physio-Medical Dispensatory: A Treatise on Theraputics, Materia Medica, and Pharmacy in Accordance with the Principals of Physiological Medication.* Cincinnati, OH, USA: W.M. H. Cook.

Wood, M. (2009). *The Earthwise Herbal- A Complete Guide to New World Medicinal Plants.* Berkeley, CA, USA: North Atlantic Books.

Wood, M. (2008). *The Earthwish Herbal- A Complete Guide to Old World Medicinal Plants.* Berkeley, CA, USA: North Atlantic Books.

Made in the USA
Lexington, KY
25 July 2015